Pain as Man's Constant Companion, f
Its Cultural, Medical and Histori(

Studies of History of Medicine, Art and Literature

Issue 49

The title illlustration shows an excerpt from a painting by Franz Skarbina with a surgical scene of the surgeon Ernst von Bergmann at the Berlin Surgical University Hospital.
Lithography, 1906. Privately owned

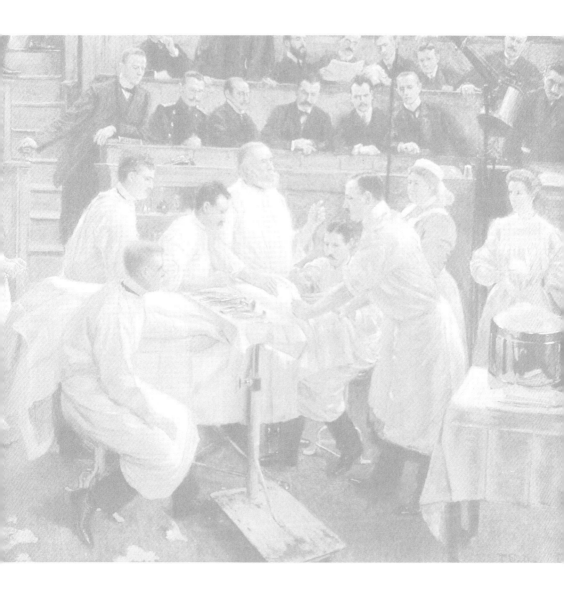

Axel Hinrich Murken

Pain as Man's Constant Companion, from Birth to Death.
Its Cultural, Medical and Historical Dimensions

Volume 1

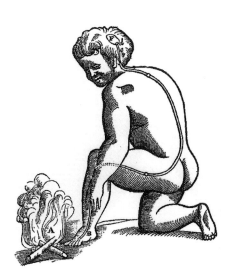

Foreword	7
Introduction	9
Pain: Man's Companion from Birth to Death	13
The First Victory - The Triumph of Anaesthesia	21
Painless Operating and Wound Healing From Drip Anaesthesia by Hand to Controlled Anaesthesia by Machine	27
Pain: Protecting and Torturing Human Life The Long Road to Understanding and Treating Pain	35
Interdisciplinary Control, Individual Treatment Old and New Concepts to Combat Pain	45
Treating Pain with Simple Healing Methods The Options of Naturopathy and Alternative Medicine	54
Proven Remedies for Pain Relief The Self-healing Powers of Human Biological Systems with the Aid of Nature's Pain Pharmacy	65
Selected Literature	76
Register of Names	84

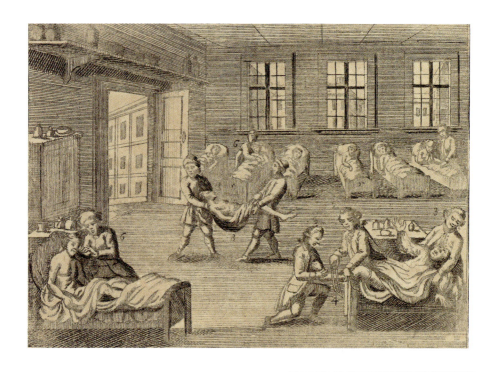

*Figure 1:
View in a patient treatment ward at Vienna General Hospital around the year 1800 with various scenes showing patient care and treatment. At the front right of the picture, a patient is shown screaming with pain as his lower leg is amputated. Lithography, around 1800.*

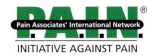

INITIATIVE AGAINST PAIN

FOREWORD

Pain. The feeling of pain, in its physical and emotional significance and scale, surpasses all other feelings that accompany man throughout his lifetime, from birth to death. No word or concept is as much associated with feelings and the soul of mankind as pain. It is encumbered with the deepest experience of the senses and emotions and can cut to the innermost core of those people who suffer from it. Moreover, it is capable of completely controlling and changing man's thinking and behaviour in incomparable ways.

European studies show that about 50 % of the adult population suffer from one or more types of pain at any given point of time. This percentage increases markedly with age. Pain is therefore a major healthcare problem in Europe. Although very few people die of pain, many die in pain and even more live in pain (EFIC's declaration, 2001).

Under the aegis of the European P.A.I.N. Initiative, projects are being assembled which will provide direct support for patients, physicians and relatives. P.A.I.N. has set itself the goal of identifying, developing and implementing practicable and practice oriented concepts for continuously improving the quality of pain management throughout Europe.

Just how pain is felt and borne is manifested completely differently, from man to man, from nation to nation, and from epoch to epoch. The intensity of pain is also assimilated in very different ways. Today, even though we already know from neurological-physiological research that special receptors (nocireceptors) are responsible for conducting pain sensations to the brain through the body's central nervous system, the phenomenon of pain still remains a puzzle. On the one hand it warns and protects us, but on the other hand it torments us and can drive us to the deepest despair.

For quite some time artists have tried, with body and soul, to depict the distress and destructive power of pain. Even though incomparable expression was captured in the late Gothic altar panels showing the torment suffered by Jesus Christ along the path to his crucifixion or in the paintings of the Christian martyrs, it was actually not until the 17th century that artists attempted for the first time to portray pain in its entire dimension. The period when artists brought their own psychosomatic feelings, their suffering and pain experience into, bear in their paintings spanned from the Baroque age to the 20th century.

For centuries doctors were helpless in the battle against pain. They could ease the sensation of pain with a few drugs, but they could not eliminate it. It was only with the discovery of nitrous oxide (laughing gas) as an anaesthetic, introduced into surgery wards in 1846, that this was expected to change. However, it was not actually until the end of the 19th century, with the discovery of aspirin, that doctors were given the first really effective medicine against pain.

Over the last fifty years, numerous pharmaceutical products and various forms of naturopathy have been introduced that promise success in the ongoing battle to conquer pain. Medical diagnosis and pain therapy offered in modern doctors' surgeries and clinics today offer many possibilities. Current holistic medicine meets the growing need in view of the worrying fact that pain and suffering have spread in almost epidemic proportions throughout the Western World. And so it seems more important than ever to establish a clear picture of the phenomenon of pain, its cultural, historical and medical significance, as well as its latest dimensions. This book is meant to be a contribution to this end and many thanks to Grünenthal for the kind support in the realisation of it.

Aachen, August 2004
Professor Axel Hinrich Murken, MD, PhD

INTRODUCTION

Since ancient times, when man first emerged from the darkness of his evolutionary history a hundred thousand years ago, he has been accompanied on his earthly journey from birth to death by pain. A highly unwelcome condition, a torment affecting his thinking, feeling and actions to a greater or lesser degree depending on its intensity. Even until relatively recent times, pain had simply to be endured as a "primeval feeling of unpleasure". For example, until the mid 19th century a surgical operation inevitably involved almost unimaginably horrendous pain (Figure 1). Naturally, man struggled against pain from the very beginning, for thousands of years. As time went on, he devised all manner of techniques to overcome this phenomenon, ranging from the use of medicinal herbs in the form of soporific sponges, opium juices and extracts of henbane and even magic and shamanistic rituals.

Even in the mythologies of antiquity and the religions of the world, the experience of suffering pain formed a focal point of legends, myths and parables permeated by feelings of guilt and expiation. The well-known Greek legend of the Titan Prometheus who because of his love of mankind, made them the gift of fire against the wishes of Zeus, the father of the gods, was punished for his disobedience by having pain inflicted upon him (Figure 20). Shackled and pierced through by a rock, he was tormented day and night by a giant eagle tearing at his liver, causing his body to writhe in unbearable pain. Even the expulsion of Adam and Eve from paradise as related to us in the Old Testament was also bound together with the curse of future pain, because it was God's judgement that in future women on earth would give birth to their children only through pain.

Only with the establishment of Western medicine by Hippocrates and his followers in the 4th century before Christ did physicians residing near the shrines dedicated to Aesculapius, the god of healing, attempt to define the phenomenon of pain, investigate it rationally and try to eliminate its causes to relieve suffering. Although no effective means were yet available, it was the fundamental principle of Hippocratic medicine that medical treatment should avoid unnecessary pain. Essentially, it should be "tuto, cito et jucunde" - rapid and not unpleasant. Yet even the most minor surgical intervention was associated with pain and fear. Pain was thus a permanent accompaniment of all surgical treatments. Only when the first anaesthetics in the form of laughing gas and other narcotic gases began to be used for operations from 1846 onwards, did the situation change to the patients' advantage.

For a long time, physicians had great difficulty in understanding how pain arises and is propagated in the human body. Why does it take such a heavy toll of the soul and spirit? Were there tiny channels conducting the pain sensation from the skin to the brain, as the philosopher René Descartes (1596-1650) believed in the 17th century? Or did it have to do with the blood which, as William Harvey (1578-1657) demonstrated in 1628, circulates throughout the body? In any event, experiments at eliminating pain by injecting opium solutions into the blood stream were performed in the mid 17th century. But, unfortunately, the unhygienic and imprecise methods used at that time tended to harm patients more than help them.

Not until the 19th century did physiologists discover the sensory mechanisms of the skin. They found receptors and special fibres that appeared to be responsible for conducting pain sensation. An even more significant advance in pain control was achieved by the pharmacist Friedrich Wilhelm Sertürner (1783-1841), who in 1806 isolated the alkaloid morphine from opium.

He thereby prepared the first effective drug to have both pain relieving and euphoric effects in man. The drug was named morphine after Morpheus, the Greek god of sleep and dreams. Even more important, however, was the development of anaesthesia which from 1846 onwards, after the first use of laughing gas (N2O) as already mentioned, soon became an indispensable part of every surgical procedure, and from 1950 onwards was established as a medical discipline in its own right.

Finally, the physicians Roland Melzack and Patrick David Wall, postulated the gate control theory, a readily understandable and practicable model of the production and duration of pain: according to this model, inhibitory mechanisms in the spinal cord (gate) and central nervous processes as control functions (control) determine the perception but also the intensity of pain. The full complexity of reactions to painful injuries gradually became understood from the 1950s onwards, thanks to increasingly sophisticated physiological and psychological research methods. It was realised that a network of psychogenic factors, constitutional features, psychosocial circumstances and sensory properties influence pain and its individual perception.

This brief review can only give a general idea of the long periods of time that were necessary during the course of thousands of years before pain came to be understood in its full implications, freed from mystical and religious notions, researched and finally successfully treated. The fact that we have only succeeded in modern times in interpreting pain as a psychosomatic, pathological phenomenon proves what a central role pain occupies in human existence. It is a phenomenon which can only be combated by an integrated, interdisciplinary approach involving physicians, psychologists and social therapists, a fact amply demonstrated by modern pain research and therapy.

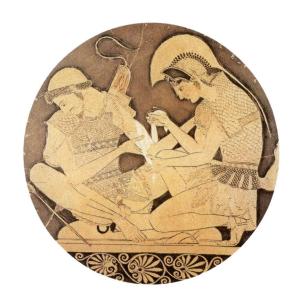

Figure 2:
The antique hero Achilles bandages his wounded companion Patrokles, who is turning away his face with a distorted expression. Red-figured bowl of Sosias. 5th century B.C.

PAIN: MAN'S COMPANION FROM BIRTH TO DEATH

It may be difficult to believe today, but as recently as five generations ago pain was simply accepted as an inevitable concomitant of life or even as a God-given fate to be borne without complaint. Like the unfortunate Job, the sick had to resign themselves to their suffering as a trial sent from above. Physicians and patients alike were exposed to an often frightful ordeal of pain and torment if surgery was necessary or suppurating wounds and cancerous tumours were consuming the body (Figure 2).

Even up to the mid 19th century, the prospect of having to enter an operating room was equivalent to being condemned to the torture chamber. The pronouncement of the famous French Professor of Medicine Alfred-Armand Velpeau (1795-1867) in his second edition of "Nouveaux elémens de médecine operative" in 1839 sums up the general attitude: "Eviter la douleur dans les opérations est une chimère." (The idea that pain can be avoided in operations is an illusion we ought to abandon.)

This was at the dawn of scientific medicine, when vapours and gases were administered experimentally to control pain during surgical procedures. The often vain attempts, by shamans, healers, wound surgeons and physicians to alleviate pain since time immemorial had now finally entered their scientific phase. As the 19th century progressed, this experimentation resulted in successful anaesthesia through the application of ether and laughing gas. The often dubious attempts, based on ancient oral and written traditions, to bring pain under control with the aid of medicinal herbs, the application of cold, hypnosis or suggestion finally became a thing of the past when nitrous oxide, laughing gas, was used for the first time in 1846.

In the ancient Greek temples dedicated to Aesculapius, three centuries before the birth of Christ, healers working in a sanatorium-like atmosphere attempted to dispel the fear and pain of those seeking a cure by performing religious rituals such as prayers of supplication, sacrifices, fasting, ablutions or processions through the sacred precincts. One of the main therapeutic approaches favoured

Figure 3:

Votive panel from the 2nd century B.C.. Aesculapius, the Greek god of healing, assisted by his daughter Hygieia, heals a sick person in his sleep.

by the disciples of Aesculapius was at least to put patients into a healing sleep by administering extracts of medicinal herbs and executing suggestive rituals (Figure 31). This concept favoured by the physicians of antiquity must often have been crowned with success, judging by the numerous votive offerings made by grateful patients to the healing deity. Many of them show the celestial

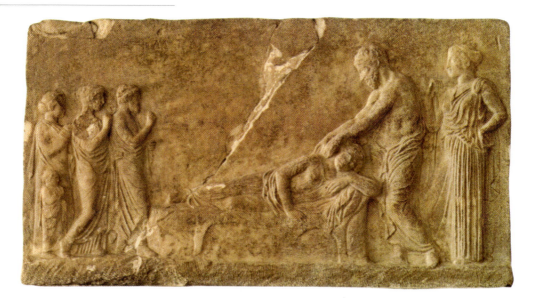

physician Aesculapius appearing to them in a dream (Figure 3 and 32).

Centuries later, at the close of the Middle Ages, artists also portrayed patients asleep during surgical procedures. Physicians had meanwhile learnt to put their patients to sleep with pain-relieving extracts of mandrake, one of the oldest medicinal plants known to man, or using "soporific sponges" (Figure 4).

Figure 4:

The mandrake plant, one of the oldest medicinal plants in the history of medicine. This old engraving shows the blossoms, fruits, leaves and roots of the mandrake. Pain-relieving extracts were obtained from the root and the fruits of mandrake, also known as mandragora.

From: M. Furlenmeier: Wunderwelt der Heilpflanzen, 3rd edition, Eltville 1980, page 113.

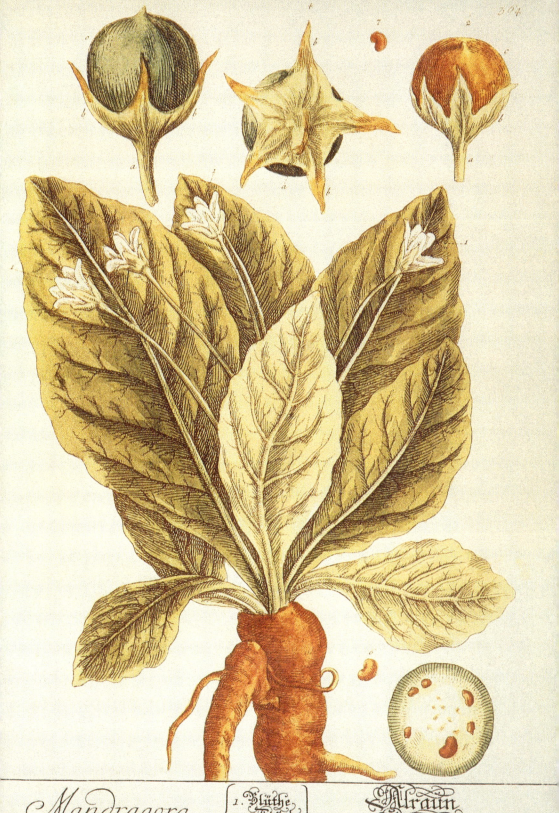

Mandragora. Alraun Alraun.

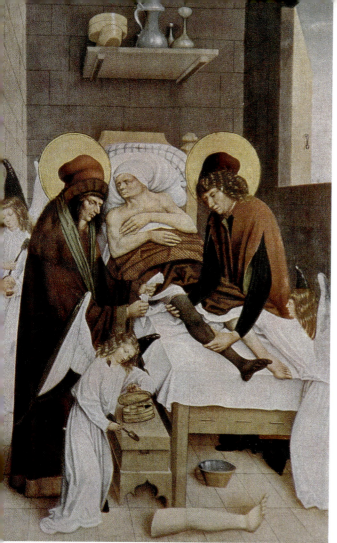

Figure 5:

The physician-saints Cosmas and Damian transplanting a dark-skinned leg, late gothic altar panel in Ditzingen dating from around 1490.

Württembergisches Landesmuseum, Stuttgart

These sponges were saturated with extracts of henbane, mandragora roots, hemlock and the juices of the poppy.

Thus treated with medicinal herbs and additionally moistened with warm water or alcohol, the sponges were held to the patient's nose and mouth. The inhaled vapours then induced sleep. Knowledge of this anaesthetic procedure makes it easier to understand the somewhat phantasmagoric scenes of surgery depicted on late gothic panel paintings, showing the two early Christian physicians Cosmas and Damian carrying out leg transplantations on sleeping patients (Figure 5).

These sponges and somnifacient extracts of Solanaceae, such as henbane or mandrake, also seem to have been used for everyday medical treatments. One typical example is the depiction of Henry II (973-1024) being cured of his bladder stone which was removed from the sleeping emperor by monks versed in the healing arts at the Benedictine Priory of Monte Cassino near Naples in the 11th century (Figure 6).

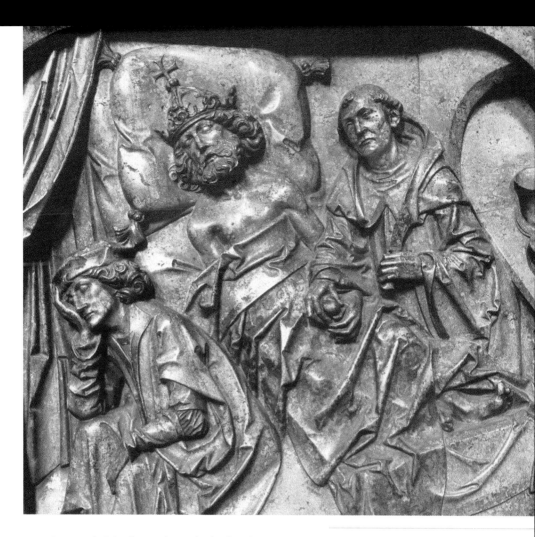

Around this time, the scholarly physician Nicolaus from the Salerno school of medicine wrote a book about antidotes, an "Antidotarium", which also included a recipe for preparing sleep-inducing sponges. These types of pain-relieving procedures are mentioned as recently as the 16th century. With the inception of the modern era, these pain-relieving practices lost importance, although they continued to be used for a long time in popular medicine as a kind of magic potion. In the 17th and 18th century, however, most

Figure 6:

Emperor Henry II having a bladder stone removed at the Italian Benedictine Monastery in Monte Cassino in 1020.

Relief on Henry II's tomb in Bamberg by Tilman Riemenschneider.

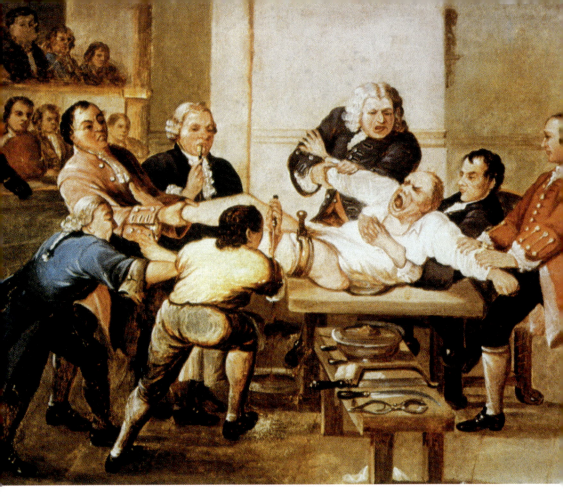

Figure 7:

Operation at St. Thomas' Hospital, London around 1750. Observed by assembled medical students, a fully-conscious patient is having a leg amputated in the operating theatre.

Illustration by an unknown painter dating from around 1750. Lithography. Private collection.

arm and leg amputations, as for example at the highly respected St. Thomas' Hospital in London, continued to be performed on conscious patients (Figure 7).

Towards the end of the 18th century, however, attempts were made to alleviate surgical pain by applications of cold and the use of suggestive hypnosis. Napoleon's famed personal physician, Jean-Dominique Larrey (1766-1842), for example, noticed during the winter campaign of 1812 that he could amputate the shattered legs of wounded soldiers on the battlefield at low

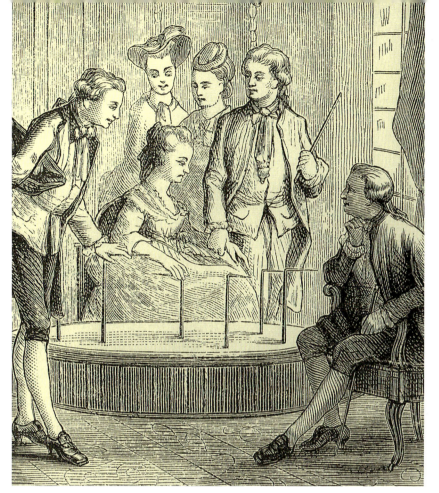

temperatures without them suffering severe pain. This method, however, did not ultimately gain acceptance.

During this same period, so-called magnetic sessions were introduced by the physician Franz Anton Mesmer (1734-1815) in Paris on the eve of the French revolution and gained great popularity (Figure 8).

At first he treated his patients, most of whom were suffering from autonomic nervous complaints, with a magnet in order to remedy the disturbed magnetic fields he believed to be present. Soon he relinquished

Figure 8:

A female patient being put into a state of artificial sleep during a magnetic therapy session based on the method of the physician Franz Anton Mesmer.

Woodcut from: Ueber Land und Meer 11 (1864).

the use of magnets and cured his clients' nervous disorders with his hands or using a mysterious "bacquet". His students succeeded in inducing "artificial sleepwalking" in patients who seemed insensitive to pain during their somnabulatory phase. But particularly the military physician Larrey, as already mentioned, like other leading physicians around 1800, were sceptical about these suggestive methods of anaesthesia.

Soon afterwards, the triumphant progress of modern inhalation anaesthesia was to begin. As early as 1774 the English natural scientist Joseph Priestley (1733-1804) prepared oxygen which was soon used in the treatment of diseases of the lung, limb pains and high blood pressure. Further experimentation with this gas inevitably followed. The English chemist Humphry Davy (1778-1829), for example, discovered nitrous oxide which he called "exhilarating or laughing gas" because of its intoxicating effect and soon considered using it as an anesthetic during operations. But almost fifty more years were to pass before anaesthesia became as taken for granted in the operating room as had previously been the screams of patients in pain.

Figure 9:

Section of a painting by Robert Hinckley: Operation under Anaesthesia, 1882.

Illustration of an excision under ether anaesthesia in Massachusetts General Hospital in Boston, 16 October 1846.

THE FIRST VICTORY - THE TRIUMPH OF ANAESTHESIA

Anaesthesia was born on 16 October 1846 in the New World in Massachusetts General Hospital in Boston where ether was first used as an anaesthetic during an operation (Figure 9). The Greek name for this volatile alcohol derivative, the vapours of which produce unconsciousness on inhalation, is "ether", which can translated as "heavenly air". During the operation, attended by several experts in the field of surgery, a tumour was painlessly

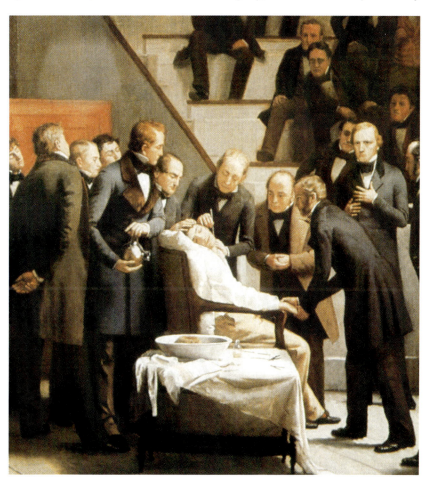

removed from the neck of a 20-year-old printer, who inhaled ether vapours prior to the operation through an inhalator.

One of the witnesses of this first painless procedure, the surgeon Henry Jacob Bigelow (1818-1890), recorded this sensational demonstration and sent his report to the American Academy of Arts and Sciences. At the same time at the end of 1846 he published it in the renowned Boston Medical and Surgical Journal under the title "Insensibility Surgical Operations Produced by Inhalation". It took just two to three months for this spectacular event from the world of medicine to reach Europe, where successful attempts at combating pain with ether were made in Paris, Bern and Erlangen. Both surgeons and obstetricians used this narcotic in the great hope of helping patients.

Nowadays the moral reasons against the use of narcotics that caused an uproar at the time might seem to be a historical curiosity. The protests stemmed particularly from the fact that since early ages of man, pain was considered to be ordained by God. For example, "Canstatt's Annals on the Progress of Medicine in all Countries" in 1847 states that "For reasons of theory, experience, morals, humanity and caution, etherisation in obstetrics is totally inadvisable".

In Germany the dedicated Berlin surgeon Johann Friedrich Dieffenbach (1792-1847) helped ether to a breakthrough in the treatment of pain in his famous book "Ether in the Treatment of Pain" in 1847. In addition to ether, chloroform was also soon to be used in surgery and obstetrics. Hardly a year after the epochal operation in Boston Central Hospital, the Scottish physician James Young Simpson (1811-1870) announced, before the Medico-Surgical Society of Edinburgh, the analgesic success of this clear liquid. It smells sweet and evaporates at room temperature. Like ether, inhalation of chloroform vapours abolishes pain sensitivity. This new anaesthetic became

Figure 10:

Illustration of an inhalator for anaesthesia using chloroform vapours, constructed by Dr John Snow.

Engraving in the London Medical Gazette, 1848.

world-famous in 1853, when no other than Queen Victoria was given chloroform by Dr John Snow (1813-1858) during the birth of her son Leopold (Figure 10).

In the following decades, ingenious surgeons constructed various inhalators for ether and chloroform vapours. The simplest medico-technical solution was invented in the 1870s in the form of a mask covering the mouth and nose, on to which ether solution was dripped and the patient inhaled the vapours. The young German physician Curt Schimmelbusch (1860-1895) constructed a mask with replaceable gauze at the Berlin University Surgical Clinic which generally became known as the Schimmelbusch mask (Figure 11).

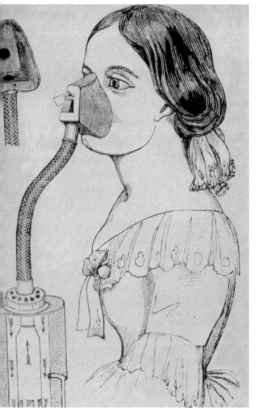

Another step in the battle against pain was infiltration anaesthesia introduced by the surgeon Carl Ludwig Schleich (1859-1922). In 1892 he used physiological saline solution with 0.1% cocaine, which was infiltrated around the operation site. This was the birth of local anaesthesia. However, the surgeons attending the annual congress of the German Surgical Society in Berlin in 1892 were at first extremely sceptical. Nevertheless, this method soon prevailed, and at the beginning of the 20th century, further improvements were made to this method by inventing synthetic substitutes and adding adrenaline to delay absorption. This hormone from the adrenal medulla was first synthesised from the ovine adrenal cortex in 1900, from which its name is derived (ad renes = at the kidneys).

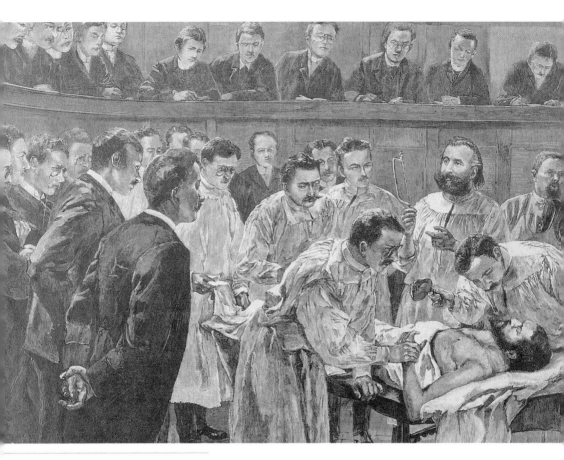

Figure 11:

View of the operating theatre of the Berlin University Surgical Hospital in 1891. The surgeon Ernst von Bergmann shortly before amputating an arm. The patient was anaesthetised using a Schimmelbusch ether mask.

Sketch by Werner Zehme, 1891.

Its great success was finally due to synthetic eucaine, and in particular novocaine, and not cocaine or other compounds. Novocaine is said to have been introduced into anaesthesia in 1905 by the chemist Alfred Einhorn (1817-1917). It was patented directly after its discovery and combined with adrenaline as a local anaesthetic. In the same year Leipzig surgeon Heinrich Braun (1862-1934) published his pioneering textbook on local anaesthesia (Figure 12).

Figure 12:

Cover of Dr Heinrich Braun's textbook: Local Anaesthesia, its Scientific Background and Practice.

Leipzig 1905.

This proposed injecting analgesics directly into nerves and the spinal cord. As early as 1898, Kiel surgeon August Bier (1861-1949) was the first to undertake injecting a cocaine solution between the lumbar vertebrae after a lumbar puncture in order to amputate a foot. Lumbar anaesthesia, which he first introduced, was then applied to the nervous system.

Virtually at the same time, barbiturates were introduced into pain therapists' armamentarium as hypnotics. Since 1875 chloral hydrate had been used as an anaesthetic in Paris, but the dose necessary proved to be too toxic and had too many side-effects. However, this paved the way for the development of other synthetic anaesthetic substrates, resulting in barbiturates derived from urea and malonic acid in 1903. Finally a barbiturate derivative called veronal was synthesised by the clinician Joseph von Mering (1849-1908) and the chemist Emil Fischer (1852-1949) which was said to have a narcotic effect and hardly any side-effects. However, it was first used surgically as a narcotic in 1932 in the form of an easy-to-handle, short-acting narcotic.

PAINLESS OPERATING AND WOUND HEALING
From Drip Anaesthesia by Hand to Controlled Anaesthesia by Machine

Anaesthesia by means of inhalation of ether or chloroform vapours through a mask, to prevent pain, became standard in all major surgical procedures from the 1870s. There were many variations in the shape of the mask, and in Germany Curt Schimmelbusch's mask was used, on to which ether or chloroform was trickled (drip method, Figure 11 and 13). However, surgeons' opinions differed as to whether the use of chloroform or ether involved life-threatening hazards for the patient. As a result of this controversial discussion, the German Surgical Society asked the famous surgeon Ernst Julius Gurlt (1825-1899) in 1890 to carry out a statistical investigation as to which anaesthetic had caused more fatalities in the past. Gurlt found that ether faired much better than chloroform, with only one death in 14,646 patients given anaesthesia. However, despite all the euphoria in the prime of anaesthesia, the opinion of the clinician Johann von Mikulicz-Radecki (1850-1905) still holds that any anaesthesia is a risk for the life and limb of the patient. In the same year (1890) the Swiss dentist Camille Redard (1841-1910) introduced ethyl chloride for local anaesthesia in dental treatment. Ethyl chloride was used until after the Second World War as a superficial anaesthetic in minor surgery.

At the time, however, attempts were being made to find new ways of achieving anaesthesia during surgery without serious side-effects. In 1875 French physician Pierre-Cyprient Oré (1828-1889) developed an anaesthetic procedure in which the anaesthetic chloral hydrate was injected directly into the blood steam intravenously. This method of general anaesthesia was extended thirty years later to the injection of ether and chloroform by the German surgeon Ludwig Burkhardt (1872-1922). Soon the new analgesic and hypnotic substance Veronal, the first barbiturate sedative, was being injected intravenously. However, it was soon discovered that

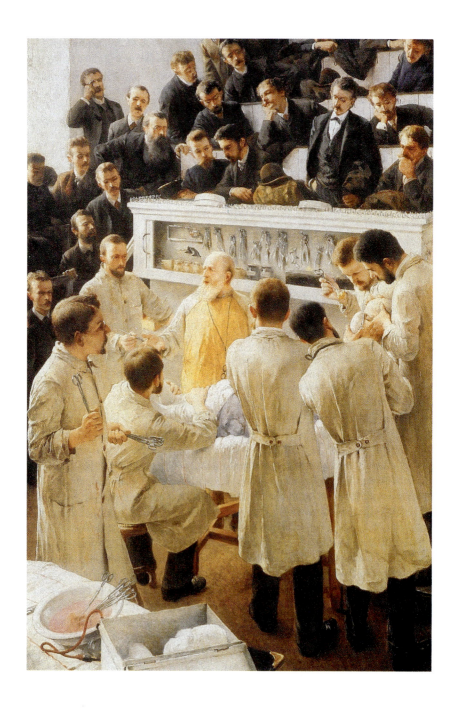

this intravenous drug was only excreted very slowly via the kidneys and was therefore very difficult to control as regards time. This problem was only solved when the pharmaceutical industry developed short-acting anaesthetics such as hexobarbital (1932) on the basis of barbituric acid, which was used to induce inhalation anaesthesia into the 1960s and proved to be a blessing to surgery.

For a time Veronal was given as a sedative on the evening before surgery in order to soothe patients' fears about the operation. Later it was succeeded by other sedatives and tranquillisers.

Although in long operations hexobarbital was excellent for the induction of anaesthesia, physicians still had to rely on ether and chloroform inhaled through a mask for analgesia. There was a considerable advance when it became possible to introduce the anaesthetics directly into the trachea via a flexible rubber tube.

The German surgeon Franz Kuhn (1866-1929) was the first to perfect this new form of intubation anaesthesia clinically. In the first decade of the 20th century in Kassel Municipal Hospital, he successfully carried out endotracheal anaesthesia which he reported in 1911 in his book (Figure 14) "Oral Intubation. A guideline on learning and performing the method illustrated by a large number of case reports" (Figure 14 and 15).

Intubation anaesthesia soon opened the gate to pulmonary surgery. In the event of respiratory arrest, the necessary physiological concentration of oxygen in the blood could still be maintained by means of a balloon on the anaesthetic machine which rhythmically pumped air into the lungs. However, for a long time the problem was that it was difficult to penetrate the narrow channel of the larynx.

The insertion of such a flexible tube into the trachea became

Figure 13:

The famous surgeon Theodor Billroth in the operating theatre of Vienna General Hospital. On the right an assistant is holding a Schimmelbusch mask over the patient's mouth on to which the anaesthetic is dripped.

Engraving after a painting of Franz Adalbert Seligmann by Richard Brend'amour 1891. From: Ueber Land und Meer 65 (1891).

surgical routine in the New World in the 1920s. Soon after 1921 the flexible tube could pass the narrow larynx, solving another problem as regards safe anaesthesia. This technique allowed effective control of the depth and duration of anaesthesia. Soon after, the first complex anaesthesia machines were developed, which supplied an oxygen/ether or chloroform mixture in a closed system by carefully controlling inhalation and expiration, i.e. inhalation of the anaesthetic by means of the exchange of carbon dioxide and oxygen. Attempts were made to avoid incidents arising from the fact that patients received too little oxygen, by developing more sophisticated machines for solid combination anaesthesia (Figure 16).

After the Second World War, muscle relaxants were also introduced into anaesthesia. The first effective muscle relaxant was curare, which inhibits the stimulation mechanism between nerves and muscle fibres. It was originally used on poisonous arrows of South American Indians and is derived from the bark of the Strychnos bush. The combination of muscle relaxants and inhalation anaesthesia from a nitrous oxide/oxygen mixture produced a more superficial gentle anaesthesia.

This development, derived from modern physiology and pharmacology, led to a new discipline in medicine shortly after the First World War: the anaesthesiology, a discipline that for a long time had been assigned to surgery. Knowledge and experience of pharmacological and physiological processes in the human body during inhalation anaesthesia rapidly increased, leading to a continuous improvement in equipment and methods. Anaesthetic journals, which first appeared in 1914, allowed for a rapid exchange of knowledge and opinions from all over the world. The journal "Der Anaesthesist" was first published in Germany in 1953, and in the same year the "German Anaesthesiology Society" was founded in Munich. Soon pain therapy and surgery without an anaesthetist was inconceivable.

Effective medicines for pain

With the beginning of modern anaesthetic procedures, pure pain treatment experienced unexpected success through new drugs.

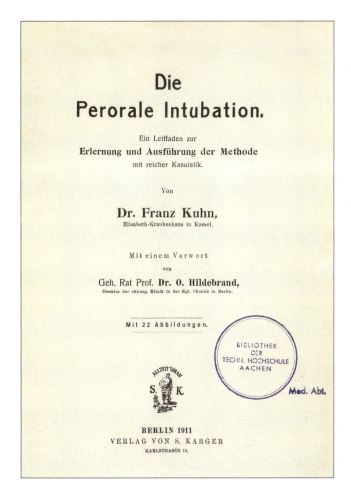

Figure 14:

Cover of the book on the new method of intubation anaesthesia by Franz Kuhn in 1911.

Two new chemical compositions of long-known pharmacological substances were undreamed-of improvements in analgesia, reducing the number of side-effects: acetylsalicylic acid known as "Aspirin" and the alkaloid of poppy juice "morphine". This was a reversion to the antique origins of medicine, in existance at the time of Hippocrates (460-375 B.C.) and his medical school, willow bark (cortex salicis) extract and the juice of the poppy, opium, were used to relieve pain, fever, and insomnia. Knowledge of these drugs, which in Greece and the Middle East were easy to obtain from the willow (Salix alba) and poppy (Papaver somniferum), remained in use in popular medicine for centuries. At the very beginning of the scientific era, the scientist Edward Stone (1702-1768) presented a chemical extract from willow bark to the learned Royal Society in London in 1763. On account of its bitter taste it was compared with cinchona bark. Therefore it was also used for febrile diseases. In the 1860s, salicylic acid achieved some

Figure 15:

Illustration of intubation anaesthesia.

In: Franz Kuhn: Oral Intubation. Berlin 1911, p. 142.

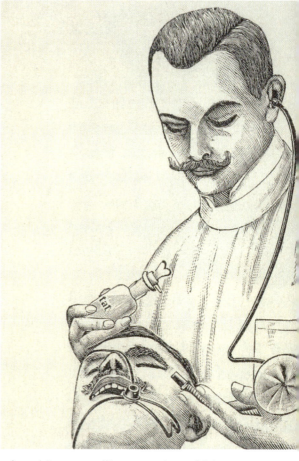

success in the treatment of rheumatic joint diseases. However, the side-effects proved too serious for the drug to be given to a rheumatism patient for long periods. Acetylation of salicylic acid and its combination with acetic acid ester by the pharmacologist Felix Hoffmann (1868-1946) produced an effective preparation which became available in the form of a white crystalline powder, which was also gentle on the stomach. After approval under the name "Aspirin" on 1 February 1899, it embarked on a triumphal march throughout the world as an analgesic and antipyretic (Figure 17).

Today, Aspirin is the No. 1 analgesic (from the Greek "an" meaning no, and "algos" meaning pain). Only since 1950 has another analgesic been on a par with it, namely paracetamol. Since 1987, these two analgesics, and other similar substances called nonsteroidal analgesics, joined those analgesics obtained from opium.

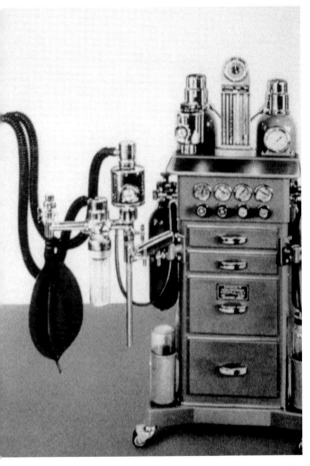

Figure 16:

The Dräger "Romulus" anaesthesia machine developed in 1951.

In: Ludwig Brandt (ed.): Illustrated History of Anaesthesia. Stuttgart 1997, p. 213.

In 1987, in a paper called "Treatment of Cancer Pain", the World Health Organisation (WHO) not only issued ten basic rules for combating pain physically and psychologically, but also devised a three-step ladder for pain therapy (Figure 18).

Another new analgesic, an opium derivative, was a drug that had become notorious since the Romance era because of the risk of addiction when taken. As early as 1806, the German pharmacist Friedrich Wilhelm Sertürner succeeded in deriving an alkaloid from opium for the fight against pain, which he called "morphine", after the Greek god Morpheus. In the 19th century, opium was found to be intoxicating and hallucinogenic. Famous writers such as Thomas De Quincey (1785-1859) ("Confessions of an English Opium-Eater") in 1822 or Charles Baudelaire (1821-1867) ("Les paradis artificiels") in 1860 described opium as a drug of bliss.

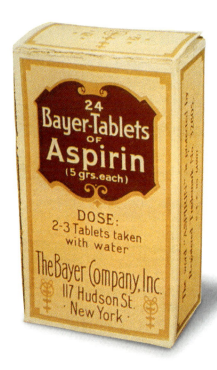

*Figure 17:
Aspirin tablets as packed for sale in American drugstores around 1910.*

In: Aspirin, a centennial drug. Leverkusen 1983, p. 36.

After the Second World War, there were legal attempts to stop open opium consumption completely, as people only saw the dangers of this drug. Only in the 1980s was opium given a new lease on life as a drug, and became integrated in pain therapy in the form of mild extracts such as codeine or concentrated substance. It was used particularly in the treatment of cancer patients or those wishing to die peacefully. Opiates and their synthetic derivatives are used clinically in different strengths for severe to very severe pain. In the meantime, research and treatment of pain have demonstrated that a multitude of factors are involved. Pain clinics and pain centres that opened after the Second World War have dedicated themselves to the interdisciplinary treatment of pain.

Figure 18:

Three-step ladder for pain therapy (WHO).

PAIN: PROTECTING AND TORTURING HUMAN LIFE
The Long Road to Understanding and Treating Pain

Pain, or pain sensation, whether due to psychological suffering or physical frailty, varies from person to person and generation to generation. In addition, pain is a complex psychosomatic process. There is no distinct transition from psychological suffering to physical pain and vice-versa. The intensity of pain sensation not only depends on individual factors, but also on social, familial and occupational circumstances. The process is altogether multifactorial.

However, as the great physician and philosopher Karl Jaspers (1883-1969) put it, there is no doubt that physical and psychological pain is a constant element of human life. The book written by the famous surgeon Ferdinand Sauerbruch (1875-1951) and the philosopher Hans Wenke (1903-1970) "Wesen und Bedeutung des Schmerzes" (Nature and Significance of Pain) (1936), which still merits reading, begins with the words: "Pain is an elementary manifestation of everything alive". Even in ancient times, it was considered that without this antagonist of health and bliss, human existence was inconceivable. Since then artists have created paintings and sculptures depicting people in great suffering, agony and pain. At the same time, however, they also wished to show how much human magnificence and tragedy can be expressed in painful suffering. This is reflected no better than in the ancient Greek Laocoon statue, the most famous example of antique art (Figure 19). With unexcelled realism, it depicts the death throes of the legendary priest and soothsayer Laocoon of Troja, with his two sons, in his excruciating physical resistance and agonising facial expression.

It was soon recognised that in human life pain is an essential element of human beings as noted above by Ferdinand Sauerbruch and has a double ambivalent significance: on the one hand it can be a valuable warning signal of an imminent or existing pathological process, demanding action to diagnose and treat the underlying disease. For this reason, in ancient times, pain was described as the "barking watchdog of health". On the other hand, this posi-

Figure 19:

The legendary Trojan priest Laocoon, who warned the Trojans of the wooden horse holding the Greek soldiers, and his sons in their desperate struggle against the deadly snakes. Apollo, the god of the sun, together with other gods, wanted to destroy Troja and so had him strangled for his betrayal.

Around 100 B.C. Vatican Museums, Rome.

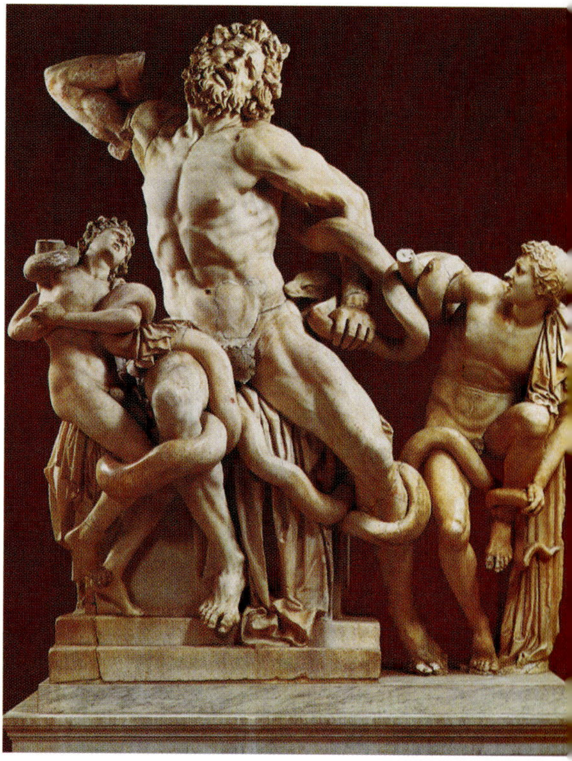

tive aspect of pain can soon reverse by becoming chronic and dissociated from the original pathological process causing it. As a result, the sufferer is no longer in a position to switch it off, like an alarm bell. A warning friend becomes an intolerable foe, and the question arises again and again: Why must people bear pain at all? The words of Karl Jaspers, as previously quoted, provide a general answer, namely people are more or less at the mercy of pain throughout their lives. For it has a general effect on the development of life.

This is confirmed by old myths and major religions that contain numerous images of it. Pain as a curse or trial of the gods even threatened and tormented Titans and Heroes. Impressive evidence of this are legends such as the

Figure 20:

A section of a painting by Jacob Jordaens: Prometheus Bound, 1645. Oil on canvas.

Wallraf-Richartz-Museum Cologne.

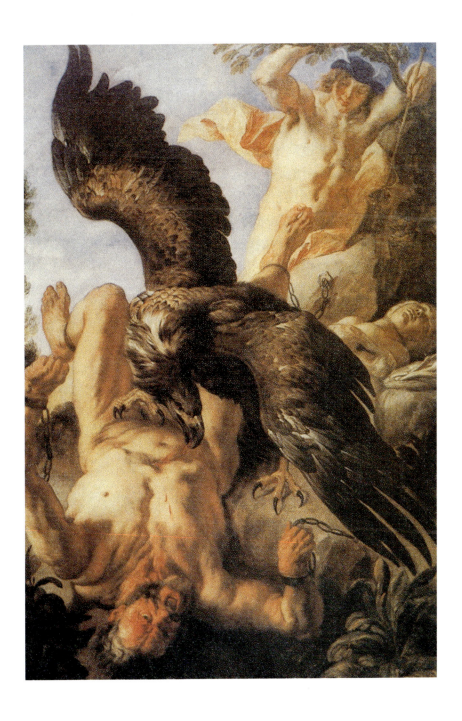

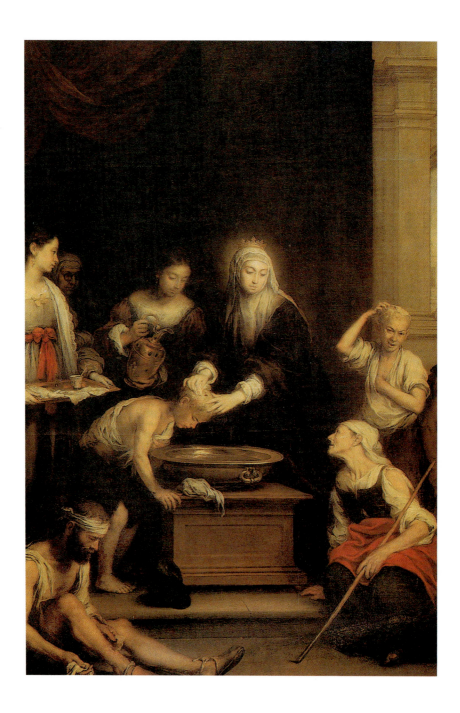

punishment of the ancient Titan Prometheus for his arrogance or the Old Testament testing of Job by God. They are infinitely embodied in art, for example the painting of Prometheus Bound by Jacob Jordaens (1593-1678) (Figure 20).

The baroque painters in the Netherlands and Spain, in particular, depicted the force and power that pain can inflict in fascinatingly exciting paintings. A number of particularly impressive testimonies were created by Spanish painters in the 17th century when the Inquisition punished dissidents and unbelievers with incredible severity. But also they show the blessing and benediction of nursing and charity. For example, the works of Bartolomeo Esteban Murillo (1617-1682) showed such scenes of charity with St. John of God or St. Elisabeth of Hungary (Figure 21).

Figure 21:

Bartolomé Esteban Murillo: St. Elisabeth of Hungary healing patients with scurf and soothing their pains.

Oil on canvas, 1667. In the church interior of La Santa Caridad Hospital in Seville (Spain).

Postcard, private collection.

For a decade now the diagnosis and treatment of chronic pain has increasingly come into focus of medical research and practice, so that now modern anaesthesia can completely control acute conditions during and after surgery. The urgency of this problem becomes evident from the fact that eight million people suffer from chronic pain that has developed from an acute event, or for no apparent reason has become a disease in its own right and simply will not cease. Its manifold causes and effects concern many disciplines of medicine. The treatment of this independent persistent pain represents an essential task for physicians in an interdisciplinary team. If chronic pain is not relieved, the brain centre may become damaged, in particular, via the nerve receptors. As a result, registration of chronic pain in the limbic system, our cerebral pain centre, intensifies, causing even more suffering. A vicious circle arises, which, if not broken, will become detrimental to the patient.

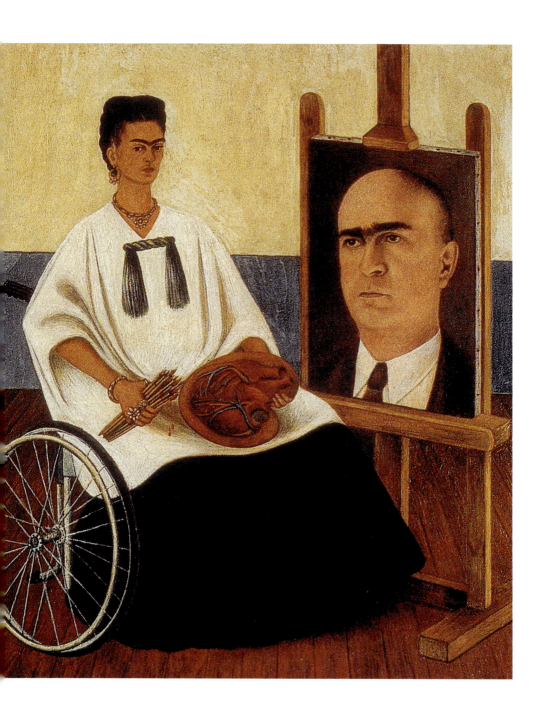

If pain has already become a disease in its own right, this is what French clinicians call a "douleur maladie". This term was coined by the great surgeon René Leriche (1879-1955) who questioned the physiological sense of pain perception in his work on pain in 1937 (Chirurgie de la Douleur, Paris 1937) amidst the euphoria of modern clinical surgery at the time, with its epochal success with the aid of anaesthesia and sterilisation. As one of the first modern clinicians, he pleaded for combating physical pain with all means available, as in his opinion this was, so to speak, a fault of nature. One argument for this procedure was that, according to early experience, local injections of narcotics had positive effects on chronic pain. In addition to Leriche, the Wroclaw surgeon Dietrich Kulenkampff (1880-1967) studied this phenomenon in the 1920s. Soon Leriche in Paris became convinced that the nervous system was responsible for the persistence of pain. He then turned to neurosurgery, a medical discipline that was still young at the time, to carry out nerve blocks with the aid of anaesthesia for exact clarification of surgical procedures. This soon produced good results.

Figure 22:

Section of a painting by Frida Kahlo: Self-portrait with the portrait of her doctor, Dr Juan Farill, 1951. Oil on hard fibre, 40 x 50 cm.

From: Helga Prignitz-Pode, Salomon Grundberg and Andrea Kettenmann (eds.): Frida Kahlo. Das Gesamtwerk. Frankfurt am Main. 1988, p. 167.

The value of a good relationship between physician and patient for combating pain, in addition to all surgical and medicinal possibilities, was demonstrated by Frida Kahlo (1910-1954), who devoted her life to combating pain, in her painting "Self-portrait with the portrait of Dr Farill" in 1951, showing her with her surgeon and general practitioner; confined to a wheelchair herself, the picture of the doctor on the easel is given the aura of an icon (Figure 22).

In her diary Frida Kahlo wrote: "I was ill for a year: 1950-1951. Seven operations on my spine. Dr Farill saved me. He returned my joie-de-vivre. ... I am not in pain. Only tired ... and of course often desperate". (Prignitz-Pode et al., Frida Kahlo, 1988, p. 260).

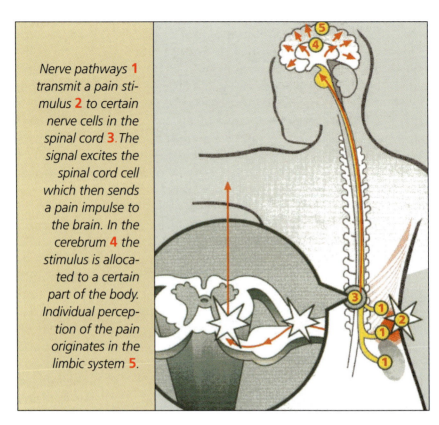

Nerve pathways 1 transmit a pain stimulus 2 to certain nerve cells in the spinal cord 3. The signal excites the spinal cord cell which then sends a pain impulse to the brain. In the cerebrum 4 the stimulus is allocated to a certain part of the body. Individual perception of the pain originates in the limbic system 5.

Medicine takes up the interdisciplinary battle against pain

Since the end of the war, medicine has shown more inclination to carry out all-embracing interdisciplinary research into the phenomenon of pain to find those structures and causes of it that are interwoven into the human body and soul. A characteristic feature of this was that in the 1980s, the American Academy of Pain Medicine was founded in the USA, which has published its own journal since 1983, "The Chemical Journal of Pain".

The first step towards interdisciplinary pain centres was made before the start of the Second World War in the famous American Mayo Clinic in Rochester where local anaesthesia was applied not only for surgery, but also for postoperative pain. One of the first to extend the range of application of local anaesthetics was the French surgeon Gaston Labat (1876-1934) in Paris, by using them not only for surgery, but also for pain in general. It was also Labat who after the First World War followed Charles Mayo's (1865-1939) call to the Mayo Clinic in Rochester, where he introduced pain therapy. In 1923 his epochal textbook "Regional Anesthesia. Its Technique and Chemical Application" was published in Philadelphia. This led the way to the first systematic nerve block with anaesthetics for pain in general. This was soon followed by information presented at congresses of the American Regional anaesthesia Society founded in 1923. First progress was made by the American anaesthetist John Joseph Bonica (1914-1994) who introduced the team approach of interdisciplinary consultation and treatment of pain patients. As early as 1947 he recognised that various problems are associated with pain and its treatment. In 1953 he published the first medical textbook on pain therapy: "The Management of Pain".

Figure 23:

The physical route of pain: from its induction by a stimulus to its perception in the brain.

Diagram in "Contra Pain". To Avoid Unnecessary Suffering. A Grünenthal Initiative. Aachen 2003, p. 8.

As a result, the first "pain clinic" was established in 1961 at Washington State University in Seattle. This was followed by similar clinical institutions in Europe and then Germany, where typical "pain centres" were established in view of the diversity of the causes and treatment of pain. Since the 1970s more intensive research than ever before has been carried out on the target sites of various medicines and therapeutic methods for pain treatment. Focus was centred on the peripheral and central nervous system and the pain centre in the brain. A diagram shows the state of the art as regards the origin of pain sensation from the external stimulus to perception (Figure 23). René Descartes had a similar notion as early as the 17th century (Figure 24). Thanks to John J. Bonica, soon called the "World Champion of Pain" the International Symposium of Pain was first held in Seattle in 1973 at which the International Association for the Study of Pain was founded. This quickly became the parent society for national associations for the study of pain, allowing the fruitful development of pain research. In Germany the German Society for the Study of Pain was founded in 1990 along with its journal "Der Schmerz".

This was followed by its own chair for pain medicine established at Aachen University Clinic in 2002. In the last decade of the 20th century there has been a profusion of new knowledge on the development, severity and diversity of pain, which will be the subject of the next chapter.

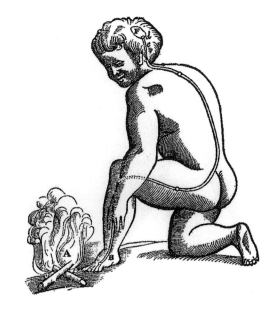

Figure 24:

Description of pain transmission by René Descartes. The heat of the fire (A) irritates the nerve endings in the foot (B) which send a pain impulse to the brain (F) to the pineal gland.

*Drawing around 1640.
From: René Descartes:
De homine. 1662 (posthum).*

INTERDISCIPLINARY CONTROL, INDIVIDUAL TREATMENT
Old and New Concepts to Combat Pain

*"As a physical sensation, it (pain) is
not merely confined to the physical domain,
but exerts effects on all levels of the soul and spirit."*
FERDINAND SAUERBRUCH AND HANS WENKE, 1936

It took a long time before the complex psychosomatic nature of pain was recognised and interdisciplinary therapeutic strategies were developed for its control. This is especially true of chronic pain, which has become a phenomenon overshadowing human enterprise in our modern era. In the USA, physicians drew attention early to the fact that chronic pain has assumed virtually epidemic proportions since the post-war period. In 1978, for example, physician Steven F. Brena titled his book dealing with the phenomenon of persisting pain: "Chronic Pain: America's Hidden Epidemic". Similarly, only recently have we begun to investigate, selectively apply and, whenever possible, combine the therapeutic resources offered by natural medicine and even homeopathy, acupuncture or esoteric healing. Depending on the severity of pain, evaluating and utilizing all aspects of the healing arts, from mainstream medicine to esoterics, should now be a self-evident approach in outpatient and inpatient pain clinics.

In the previous chapters we described how pain was suffered and endured differently from one historical epoch to the next and how these differences still persist today. Age, sex, social status or education, but also the history of human society as a whole, have to be taken into account when considering the intensity of pain, as does individual sensitivity, which can differ radically from one patient to the next with the same surgical procedure, similar joint diseases or an attack of migraine (Figure 25).

Not without reason do we tend to speak of sensitive and insensitive patients. This great variability in pain sensitivity, which depends on a multiplicity of factors, is usually subsumed under the general term "pain tolerance". But even the word "pain" originally encompassed the entire gamut of physical and mental suffering to which humans are susceptible. In contrast, the Middle High German word "Pein" originally described only physical pain. In the

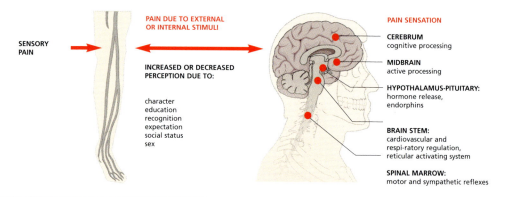

Figure 25: Pain stimulus processing.

English language, this old Germanic word eventually evolved into "pain", which includes both physical and psychological distress. The complexity and heterogeneity of the discomforts induced by pain stimuli were analyzed in detail, probably for the first time, by the physician Alfred Goldscheider (1858-1935) in his treatise "The Problem of Pain" (1920) – a work still well worth reading (Figure 26).

Although ancient Greek had several words to describe pain, as a means of distinguishing between sorrow, distress, physical complaints such as algos and algia (= physical pain) or algesis (= emotional pain) or spasmos (= seizure), a more precise diagnostic differentiation of pain only became possible with the advent of the natural sciences. From the 18th century onwards, medical researchers initially devoted themselves to studying the structure and function of the nerves after they had been characterized by the anatomist Andreas Vesal (1514-1564) in 1543. The inspired physiologist and anatomist Albrecht von Haller (1708-1777), as Professor of Medicine in Göttingen, was able to demonstrate experimentally in the mid 18th century that only the nerves can feel, transmit sensations, and cause the muscles to contract. They have the capacity of "sensitivity" and "irritability". Three generations later, clinical dermatologists and neurologists began to examine the nerve endings on the skin, the nociceptors (nocere, Latin = harm), sensors with the specific ability to elicit feelings of pain in the human brain. It is now believed that the pain thresholds which report the pain inducing stimulus hardly differ between individuals. In contrast, "pain tolerance" as mentioned before suggests a very heterogeneous range of pain experience. Modern neurophysiology has now shown that human innervation interconnects all parts of the body like a complex network of electrical circuits. The external stimuli travel from the nerve endings through the sensory nerves (neurons) to the eye, ear, nose or skin in the form of electrical currents. Simultaneously, they travel through the spine to the brain. Neurons consist of three main parts: 1) cell body, 2) an axial cylinder (axon) and 3) a branched network (dendrites) (Figure 27).

Impulses generated by chemical metabolic processes are fed into this conduction network flowing from the periphery by sensory neurons to the centre of the brain, but also from there to the muscles, internal organs and skin to induce by motor neurons reactions such as muscle tension, peristaltic movements or reddening of the skin. The previous chapter contained a schematic diagram illustrating in simplified form the pathway followed by a receptor mediated impulse from the back through the spinal marrow to the brain by Descartes (Figure 24).

The processes involved are naturally much more complex than can be shown in any schematic diagram, since the impulses

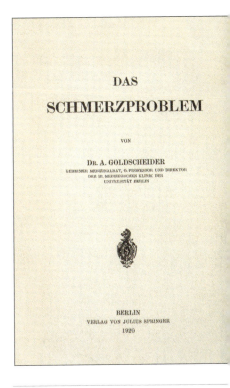

Figure 26:

One of the first scientific books on the phenomenon of pain. Title page by: Alfred Goldscheider: Das Schmerzproblem [The Problem of Pain]. Berlin 1920.

passing between the central control site in the brain and the tactile and sensory endings are in a state of permanent exchange with the associated cell bodies in the different parts of the body. The comparison with a power supply network also makes it clear why the cells and fibres of the nervous system become increasingly thicker as they travel through the spinal marrow in the vertebral canal and onwards to the brain. It is indeed like an electrical conduction system with a central switching and metering unit from which

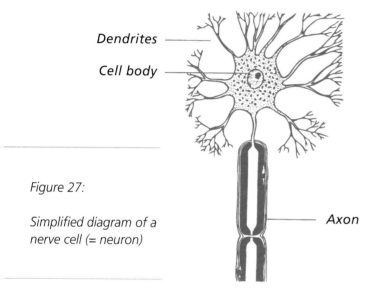

Figure 27:

Simplified diagram of a nerve cell (= neuron)

numerous supply lines travel from the kitchen to the bedroom, from the basement to the loft and back again (Figure 25 and 28).

In outlining the anatomical and physiological principles necessary for an understanding of the nature of pain conduction, it is important to realize that the overall human nervous system is made up of three different interacting circuits:

1. the network of nerves independent of our will which controls

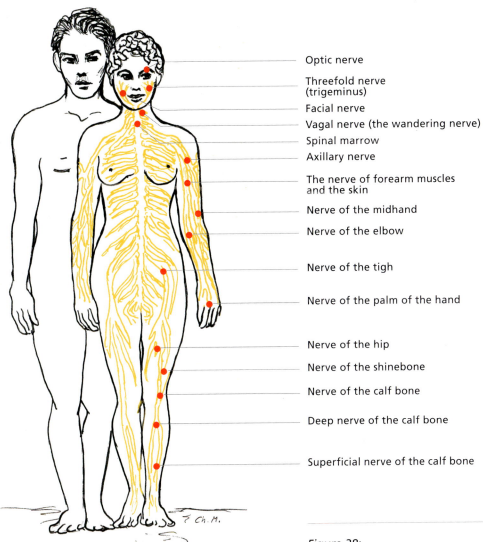

- Optic nerve
- Threefold nerve (trigeminus)
- Facial nerve
- Vagal nerve (the wandering nerve)
- Spinal marrow
- Axillary nerve
- The nerve of forearm muscles and the skin
- Nerve of the midhand
- Nerve of the elbow
- Nerve of the tigh
- Nerve of the palm of the hand
- Nerve of the hip
- Nerve of the shinebone
- Nerve of the calf bone
- Deep nerve of the calf bone
- Superficial nerve of the calf bone

Figure 28:

Locations of the individual nerves with their sensors (nociceptors) at the nerve endings.

respiration, sleep or digestion: the autonomous nervous system

2. the bundle of nerves permeating the muscles which make it possible for us to walk,

stand, sit, chew, etc., and is subject to our will: the motor nervous system

3. the nerves which conduct our feelings, thoughts and actions: the sensory nervous system

These three nervous systems, although functioning independently of each other, are almost inextricably interlinked, a fact which becomes especially clear in situations of stress, shock or grief. While 20th century neurophysiologists have obtained increasingly impressive research results, and have been able to elucidate and understand pain processes with unprecedented clarity through cooperation with histologists, neurologists and physiologists, the efforts of physicians to differentiate degrees of pain intensity, as a basis for elaborating selective therapeutic approaches, have not been conspicuously successful because biomedical knowledge alone is insufficient for this purpose. After the post-war period, it was first attempted to establish scales indicating the intensity of pain. In 1952, American pain researcher James D. Hardy, working together with other medical experts, postulated a gradation of pain intensity from 1 to 21: "There are a limited number of just noticeable differences in pain intensity, approximately 21 from threshold (pain) to maximum" (Hardy et al., 1952, page 380). Based on this system, a more easily-manageable scale, comprising ten different degrees of pain, can be postulated:

Definition of pain sensation in pain gradations from 1 to 10:
Scale describing pain sensation (according to James D. Hardy and Heinrich Felix Anschütz).

1. Hardly perceptible pain, with little effect on general well-being. The stimulus has just exceeded the pain threshold.

2. Pain that can still be mentally suppressed, but slight discomfort is present.

3. Pain which can no longer be deliberately compensated, but nevertheless does not greatly affect activities of daily life.

4. Pain which begins to bother the subject, but can still be overcome or tolerated without treatment.

5. Pain which noticeably affects daily activities and work and is continuously present.

6. Severe pain giving rise to defensive reactions. The painful part of the body or extremity assumes a relieving posture.

7. Pain experienced as intense. It pushes all actions and activities into the background.

8. Very intense pain. The perception of this degree of pain impairs all activities, including vital activities such as eating, drinking or sleeping.

9. The pain is scarcely tolerable. Experiencing this degree of pain intensity eclipses everything else and leaves hardly any scope for thought and action.

10. No longer tolerable pain. The sufferer can no longer stand the pain physically or emotionally. Mortal fear, panic and the wish to die.

Although distinguishing between different pain intensities may be difficult, a pain rating scale is a useful tool for the effective treatment of pain insofar as it allows the appropriate form of medical management to be selected and defined more accurately. Despite the substantial advances achieved by scientific medicine by using drugs to treat pain – the analgesics – (from the ancient Greek an = negation, algos = pain), it is well known that every pill can have harmful side effects. A causal therapy for this psychometric phenomenon has therefore yet to be discovered.

Summarising, we can conclude that:

1. the perception of pain is not exclusively a biochemical process,

2. the phenomenon of chronic pain has been given little attention in the history of medicine,

3. the perception and toleration of pain depends on numerous factors such as individual, social, cultural attributes or age.

Holistic methods enhance the treatment of pain to a previously unsuspected degree:

One of the previous chapters described today's conventional three-step system for the pharmacologic treatment of pain (Figure 18, page 34). It ranges from the non-opiate drug substances aspirin and paracetamol through the more potent action of the newer non-steroidal antirheumatics like ibuprofen, diclofenac, indomethacin or naproxen, the mild opiates (codeine) up to the "big gun" of the potent opiate morphine. This is the standard approach offered by mainstream medicine, but none of these therapies are free from side effects. For the milder degrees of pain, therefore, holistic forms of therapy as offered by natural medicine or other alternative therapeutic modalities should be considered. It is now a standard item on the agenda to increasingly resort to naturopathic remedies as valuable concomitants or even substitutes for conventional pharmacological therapy.

Essentially, this category includes all non-medicinal and non-surgical treatments, such as gymnastics, active or passive physiotherapy or the now very prevalent practice of Eastern esoteric with its meditative, behavioural and movement rituals. These multi-faceted forms of treatment attuned to both body and soul, which invariably take into account the psychosomatic processes occurring in the human body during pain which are different from those that occur in all other illnesses, seem almost limitless in their variety. It has been known since ancient times that the care and attention

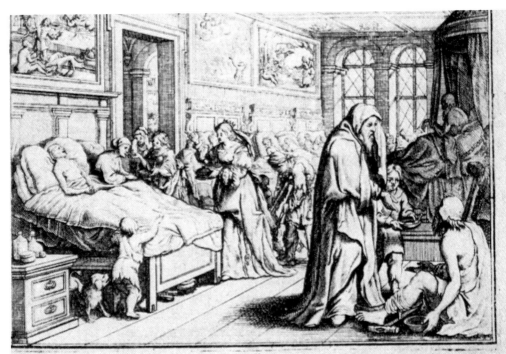

devoted to the patient either by the physician or visiting relatives and also religious belief can also help alleviate pain (Figure 29). This is the starting point for long-term, intensive, passive and active mobilisation therapies and programmes of psychotherapy extending over several years.

Figure 29:

View of an infirmary room in the Baroque period. Copperplate engraving by Abraham Hogenberg, about 1640. The scene bears the commentary: "Gladly visit the patient in his suffering and pain, then feelest thou, when sick, God's mercy in your heart".

TREATING PAIN WITH SIMPLE HEALING METHODS
The Options of Naturopathy and Alternative Medicine

> *I feel that the basis of future medicine lies in combining exact research with the preventive and healing efforts of naturopathy.*
> ALFRED BRAUCHLE, 1935

Since ancient times, man has tried to combat pain with natural healing methods. Therapeutic options for all types of pain ranged from suggestive methods, dietetic procedures and herbal therapies to fasting, balneotherapy, and the mud baths from the Stone Age to the great civilisations 5,000 years B.C.. Experience has more or less shown that man has a natural, innate, certain and correct behaviour in maintaining and fortifying his health and combating painful diseases.

These are self-healing forces that no one doubts any more. Not only prehistoric healers and the high priest physicians of the Babylonian civilisation in Mesopotamia acquired the knowledge and trust in the body's instinctive wisdom, obtained from experience, the legendary Greek physician Hippocrates with his medical school did so too, by trying to strengthen their patients' natural defences. Taking into consideration the patient's history and an exact diagnosis, treatment and prognosis, they placed great store in such alternative healing methods and concrete medical actions. A famous German physician, Alfred Brauchle (1898-1964), who encouraged naturopathy in the 1930s, mentioned in a conversation with the internal specialist Louis Radcliffe Grote: "Naturopathy claims to be the continuation of a long-gone medicine that was once considered to be conventional." (Louis Radcliffe Grote and Alfred Brauchle: Gespräche über Schulmedizin und Naturheilkunde. Leipzig 1935, p.16).

Treatment of Diseases and Pain in Ancient Times

Brauchle correctly followed on from the medicine of the adherents of Hippocrates who created a scientific basis for their medical profession 400 years B.C. at the religious sites of the Greek god of medicine Asklepios. For the first time in the history of medicine and culture they combined naturopathy and conventional medicine as a matter of course. At the time the Asklepiads, as doctors were called in the Asklepieia of ancient Greece, combined the common healing methods of suggestion and meditation known from ancient shamans together with hypnotherapy and herbal therapy in order to forftify health and heal painful symptoms of all disciplines. In the process, the patient's belief in the healing powers of the healer, whether priest or a pupil of Hippocrates, and his prescriptions, were of decisive importance for the success of the pain-relieving cure.

Today, this phenomenon appropriately described by the common saying "Faith can move mountains", is generally recognised thanks to the research of the Boston physician Herbert Benson, whose book "Timeless Healing: The Power and Biology of Belief" (1996) was also a best seller in Germany. Using this holistic, mind-body method we stimulate the patients' natural defences. As immunologists say, we strengthen our immune system. The fact that prehistoric medicine men and shamans made specific use of this method can be gleaned from their flashy clothing adorned with terrifying attributes and from their magic rituals. The best example of these early suggestive components of healing is a Palaeolithic rock painting in the cave of Lascaux in Montignac in the South of France. It shows a medicine man in the frightening disguise of a stag (Figure 30).

Such fantastic costumes of the healer, which were particularly common for shamans in the Siberian tundra even in pre-Christian times, intensified the healing effect of natural prescriptions similar to that of a placebo. In this way aromatic oils, extracts or infusions of medicinal herbs such as nettles, camomile or Saint-John's Wort, and juices from the opium during magic rituals were

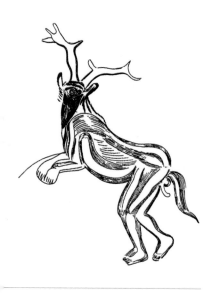

Figure 30:

Picture of a Stone Age medicine man wearing a stag's coat. With the stag's antlers and long beard, he also assumed the strength of the mighty beast of the forest.

From a Palaeolithic rock painting in the cave of Lascaux (South of France). Around 10,000 B.C..

considerably more effective.

Such a close entwinement of naturopathic and suggestive, magic healing methods also developed in the ancient temple and cult sites dedicated to the Greek god of medicine, Asklepios, and the superior Apollo since the 4th century B.C. throughout in the ancient world.

A patient who visited the Asklepios temple in Pergamon, now called Bergama, founded about 280 B.C., was accommodated in the best hygienic and climatic conditions in long corridors with open, columned halls surrounding the generously laid out area.

The Asklepieion centre was the Temple of Apollo who was worshipped as a healing and sun god (Figure 31). Pilgrims in search of healing used to stay for several days in the temple area which, with its colonades, amphitheatre and library, not only catered for entertainment and education, but also completely rounded off the psychosomatic healing concept.

The Asklepiads, Asklepios' disciples, whose art of healing was passed on from generation to generation in ancient Greek physicians' families, treated those searching for healing in ancient times with the legendary hypnotherapy and also, as part of their holistic medicine, with fasting and balneotherapy. According to legend, the god of medicine, Asklepios, appeared personally to the patients in their dreams to provide dietetic instructions for body and soul and therapeutic intervention. Aesculapian snakes, which were kept in the Asklepieia, crawled over the half-naked bodies of sick people whilst asleep (Figure 31).

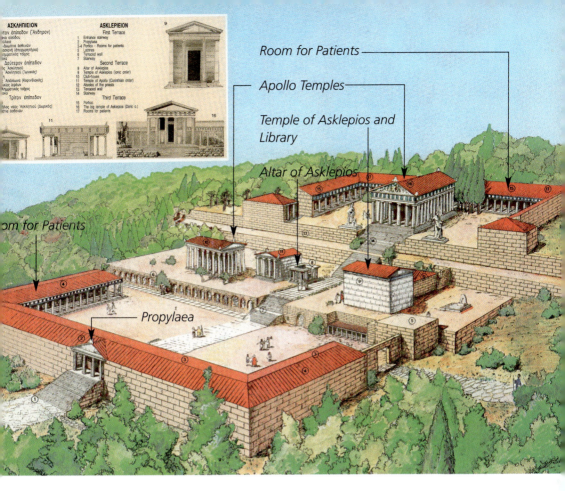

We can compare the art of healing carried out in the Askelpieia with today's rehabilitation in convalescent hospitals with the aim of reinforcing our own defences and encouraging patients to lead a balanced way of life. This method of healing is fundamentally the basis of the body and mind movement of the clinician Herbert Benson, which reactivates the old body-soul therapeutic concept with its holism. Increasingly since the seventies there has been a tendency in pain therapy to combine conventional methods with the whole spectrum of naturotherapy

Figure 31:

Asklepieion of Kos founded in the 4th century B.C. on the west slope of the mountain Dikaios. Steel engraving around 1910 from a drawing by the German archeologist Rudolf Herzog showing a reconstruction from excavations.

Privately owned.

and alternative methods to form comprehensive treatment. The fact that such integrative therapies were carried out very successfully in the ancient Asklepieia over 2000 years ago can be seen from the numerous ancient votive tablets and holy inscriptions

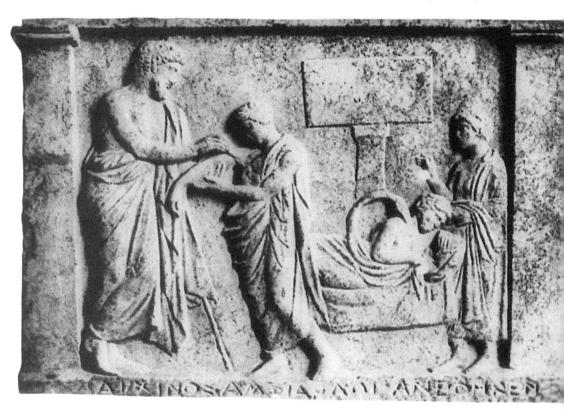

donated by grateful patients. Impressive votive tablets which archaeologists have excavated in the Asklepieia are evidence of the medical significance of this early psychosomatic form of healing (Figure 3 and 32).

The development of the Asklepieia as a type of sanatorium in the ancient world originally dates back to mythology which addresses the imaginative powers in humans and the Christian history of salvation. Later Asklepios is said to have been a popular physician in Thessalia in early Greek history before he became the principal god of medicine in the heaven of Olympus. In the 4th century, the religious cult around this legendary figure spread throughout the Mediterranean with the temple medicine in the Asklepieia named after him. Hippocrates, born 460 B.C. on the edge of the old Asklepieion of the island of Kos not far from the Turkish coast, was familiar from youth onwards with the psychosomatic medicine practised, because his forefathers had been physicians there for generations.

Figure 32:
Relief on a marbled votive stone (around 400 B.C.) from the amphiareion in Oropos (Attika in Greece). The picture shows Amphiaros worshipped as a god of healing treating a patient with an injured shoulder. Far right there is the cured patient Archinos pointing to the relief plaque dedicated by him. Archaeological National Museum, Athens.

From ancient medicine and its physicians, we learn that medicine based on rationale can be brilliantly linked with alternative healing methods which cannot be explained by our five senses. The "Corpus Hippocraticum", originating in the 4th and 3rd centuries B.C., mentioned an empirical medicine which worked with rational therapies, but also endeavoured to reinforce the patients' psychosomatic defence mechanisms by addressing their reason and by means of suggestive rituals. From an early stage, it was obvious that scientific medicine based on rational therapies may go hand in hand with alternative treatment from suggestive procedures, to hydrotherapy to diet.

From the ancient art of healing to today's healing methods

Today, in the case of chronic pain and sometimes pain which is very difficult to locate, the almost banal American maxim "Think positive" should be always taken into account, as it was in days gone by. The aim is to stimulate self-healing powers via human reasoning and to awake the "physician in us". We can differentiate this simple auto-suggestive therapy hidden in these familiar words even more in order to defend our own bodies as affected by pain:

1. "I have got the powers of healing within me."
2. "I believe in my healing."
3. "I am physically and mentally strong enough to overcome my painful disease."
4. "With my positive thinking I control my body."

According to reports and stories of healthy and also sick people who do look on the bright side, there is apparently a healing pain-relieving effect coupled with new life energy even in cases of severe cancer with its very painful symptoms. In the process, as we know today, emotional spheres are addressed which reinforce the inner biochemical defence mechanisms and make the physiological barrier impermeable to pain so that it is perceived less consciously. Several years ago, research was started in this subdiscipline of immunology which affects the strong network between body and soul. In hospitals the term "psychoneuroimmunology" has become common.

This involves old and new relaxation techniques, such as anti-stress programmes, yoga, meditation, massage, fitness training and much more. As part of such relaxation measures, it is also important to pinpoint your own pain, to realise it yourself and describe it in words. This is also called "visualisation" of the pain. In the meantime medical science is convinced by the idea of the "gate control theory", which assumes that the human psyche has a control function on pain perception, that pain sensations such as feeling, hearing and tasting are perceptions in their own right.

This concurs with the conviction expressed even by serious clinicians that our brain can suppress pain. Indian fakirs are examples of this voluntary pain suppression. In their religious yearning for salvation by means of self-castigation and renunciation, they rest naked on a bed of nails (Figure 33).

Therefore, visualisation techniques are also beneficial, because if we visualise our painful suffering then we can use our consciousness to combat our pain perception better. For example, if we per-

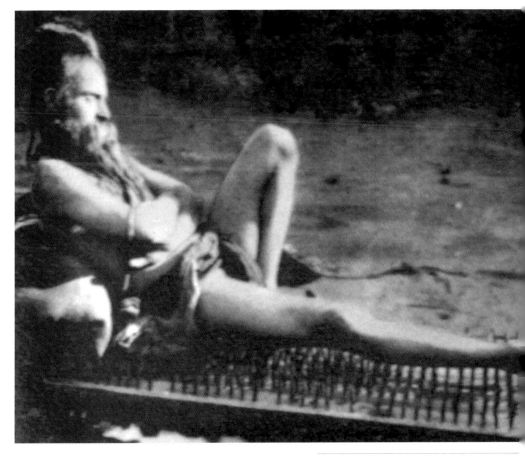

ceive the painful destruction of our body by cancer or injury as a lion, then we can try to keep it in check. Or if we perceive the pain as a knife, a sharp stone or a rock, then the obvious thing is to resist it by alienating this foreign body. This leads to the notion of armouring the skin, removing the stone or pushing away the rock.

Figure 33:

An Indian fakir sleeping on a bed of nails.

Photograph around 1960.

Some paintings of the French artist Henri Rousseau (1844-1910), one of the great post-impressionists, reflect very well such subconscious behaviour against impending suffering with pictures of dreaming women together with terrifying lions. Dangers perceived in a daze appearing in the form of the lion, are tamed in a world of make-believe safety. In this way Henri Rousseau's picture "The Dream" dated 1910 is fascinating for its composure and peace depicting a woman lying naked on a sofa looking at a lion coming out of the jungle. By gesticulating her extended arm and hand she brings the lion to a halt with an almost hypnotic power.

Figure 34:

An artistic illustration of how sympathy and charity, emotional and physical affection can alleviate emotional suffering and physical pain.

Christa Murken:
Affection, 2001.
Oil on canvas, 95 x 120 cm.

In the great religions such as Hinduism, Buddhism and Christianity the self-healing regulation mechanisms in humans are enhanced by various rituals such as prayer, meditation and yoga. Meditation resembles the process of dreaming and light sleep, the curative effect of which ancient physicians also exploited in their hypnotherapy. Nowadays meditation is an integral part of alternative methods of healing and psychotherapies. It provides relaxation by giving physical and inner peace.

This is also the purpose of post-Sigmund Freud (1856-1939) psychotherapy to recognise and solve problems leading to worries and suffering in group or face-to-face discussion. Such psychic and meditative procedures have been complemented for a decade by mind and body medicine.

These completely natural methods of healing from person to person are based on the immediate attention of a psychologically healthy person to a patient suffering from pain. This applies in particular to the "healing method" advocated for some time. Patients are treated suggestively in this process by a healer standing in close proximity in the form of concentrated telepathy and various touching techniques to arouse their natural defences and healing powers. In this way healing power is transferred from person to person which combines with the patient's own healing tendencies.

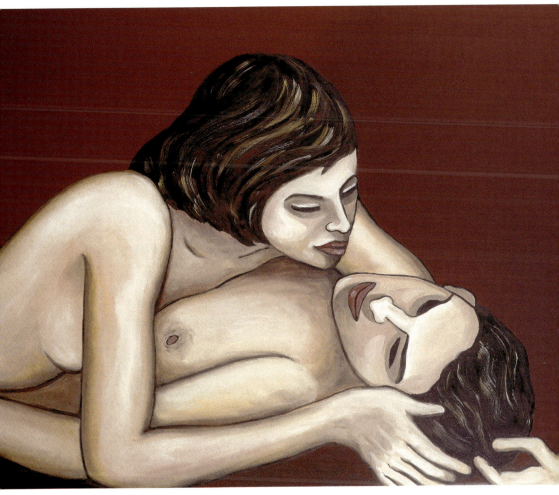

In the meantime such simple "attention" therapies are associated with "therapeutic touch" methods. This involves touching and stroking the patients and giving them familiar music to listen to and fragrances to inhale. In extreme cases even the patients' partners are allowed to lie in bed with them to provide intimate affection, warmth and love. This has been used particularly in patients who have been in a coma for a long time and in people suffering from apallic syndrome and it promises success (Figure 34). This is impressively expressed in the Spanish film "Hable con ella" (2001) ("Speak to Her") by Pedro Almodovar, where a comatose woman, cared for day and night by a male nurse who loves her, wakes up after many years on the birth of their child, fully recovered. Such simple methods of healing which are based particularly on suggestion, may be intensified by herbal therapy. This will be the subject of the next chapter.

Figure 35:

Illustration of the field camomile.

The white-yellow flower buds contain oil of camomile.
It is antispasmodic, analgesic, and diaphoretic.

From: Dioskurides: Herbal Book. German translation by Petrus Uffenbach. Frankfurt am Main 1610, page 234.

PROVEN REMEDIES FOR PAIN RELIEF
The Self-healing Powers of Human Biological Systems with the Aid of Nature's Pain Pharmacy

For thousands of years in the past, up to the beginning of the 20th century, the practice of medicine consisted, for the most part, in the use of extracts and essences from medicinal plants, in addition to psychosomatic medicine and the surgical treatment of external wounds. Already in the first century AD, the Roman military physician Dioskurides, from Greece, presented an extensive medicinal treasury, of over 600 medicinal plants, in which he recommended natural medicine for the treatment of the most prevalent illnesses. In the Middle Ages, it was the famous nun, Hildegard von Bingen (1098-1179), an early natural scientist, who dedicated her entire life to the study of medicinal herbs. She wrote learned treatises on natural history and healing with natural medicine, such as the book "Physica", which achieved great acclaim in the 13th century. In her theory on natural medicine, she viewed sick people as a physical-spiritual unit, as Hippocrates also did in ancient times, and believed that one must heal them in a comprehensive manner, i.e., in their entirety. In the 16th century, a number of noteworthy physicians and pharmacists laid the foundations for today's phytotherapy, building on the wealth of herbal medicine studies and experience of Dioskurides, who can also be described as the first pharmacologist in world culture. Thus, the physician Petrus Uffenbach of Frankfurt am Main, published a reworked and expanded version of the "Dioskurides" in 1610, the German text of which was accompanied by outstanding plant illustrations and explanations. The field camomile from which tea is extracted, as originally illustrated in this work, is still an essential element in any well-stocked medicine cabinet (Figure 35).

Leonhard Fuchs (1501-1566) pioneered some work before that in extracting medicines from nature with his "New Herbal Book" published in 1543. The medicinal plants mentioned in Fuchs' herbal textbook were pictured in a very modern and realistic way and their uses and applications were explained in such great detail that even a layman could put them into practice.

Pietro Andrea Matthioli (1500-1577) added, with his printed "Herbal Book" of nearly 500 pages in 1626, a further naturopathic compendium (Figure 36).

Figure 36:

Title page of "Herbal Book" by Pietro Andrea Matthioli surrounded by symbolic illustrations. They allude to the wealth of experience of ancient physicians and the "Pharmacy of Nature". Published by the Classicist and Physician Joachim Camerarius from Nürnberg. Frankfurt am Main 1626.

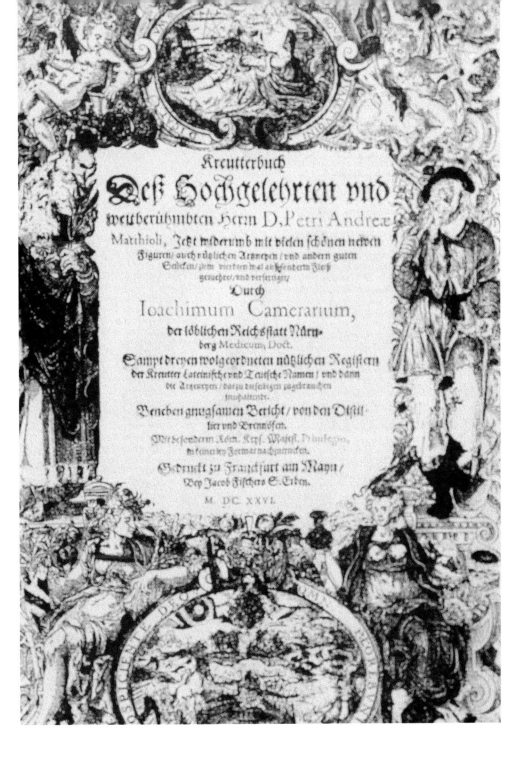

One can say with justification that, until the beginning of the era of synthetic medicines in the 20th century, that phytotherapy, the use of various elements of medicinal plants, together with psychosomatic measures, promised the most effective cure. Some medicinal plants which are still used to relieve pain today are listed here as examples:

Medicinal Herbs

Balsam
Aromatic mixture of resins and ethereal oils from numerous trees and shrubs as a base for external use and application

Eucalyptus (Eucalyptus globulus)
Extracts from leaves

Willow (Salix alba)
Extract from bark juices (salicylic acid, also contained in aspirin)

Juniper Berry (Juniperus communis) as a puree or jam.

Hawthorn (Crataegus oxycantha)
Flowers and fruit

Mandrake (Alraune)
(Nightshade family) Extracts from leaves, flowers and roots

Valerian (Valeriana officinalis)
As a brew or tincture

Herbal Analgesics

Ethereal oils from tree bark and essences from medicinal herbs that have a pain-relieving effect:

Effect
Relieves joint pain and relaxes abdominal complaints.
Germicidal, reduces swelling, soothing effect. Especially in the ears, nose and throat.
Analgesic, provides physical and emotional relaxation.
Used in gout and rheumatism as well as infections and colic.
Relieves joint pain and toothache, strengthens the heart. Lessens severity of heart attacks.
Since ancient times, extracts from the mandrake plant used as an analgesic and soporific agent.
Eases colic, sedative and soporific agent.

continued next page

Medicinal Herb
Bearberry (Arctostaphylos uva-ursi) (Evergreen shrub) leaves used for brewing tea
Camomile (Matricaria chamomilla) One species is known as the mother herb oil, powder, or as a wine or tea additive.
St John's Wort (Hypericum perforatum) Used often as a tea brew

The aim of this chapter is merely to give a brief overview on the multitude of trees, bushes, shrubs and flowers growing in forests, fields and meadows, from which herbal medicines can be extracted to help reduce acute and chronic suffering. With these herbal medicines we can dampen the effects of pain, anxiety and restlessness and sometimes, even eliminate them entirely. The leaves, flowers, bark and roots were used in the past, just as we use them today, in the most varying ways, to prepare medications for internal and external use.

It is important to mention, after all that has been said, that the use of natural herbal medicines, as well as alternative healing methods such as meditation, suggestion, yoga, massage, physical fitness training, or the "laying on of hands" must be seen as a means of self-help. These self-help methods can be utilised to take advantage of the inherent healing powers of nature. The aim of this is to rectify the balance between spirit, soul and body. The link between these three basic constants of our biological systems can be easily demonstrated using the shape of a triangle (Figure 37).

Effect

Leaves used for brewing tea. Heals urinary and bladder infections.

Reduces inflammation, cramps, pain-relieving. Relieves migraine pain. Stills painful lower abdominal conditions.

Relaxing, sedative. Soothes wound and scar pain. Lessens depression and colic.

Imagine this triangle suspended like a swing. In this way, it is easy to see that an imbalance results in a feeling of discomfort, which in turn lowers the pain threshold and pain is felt more easily.

The therapies described here from naturopathy to esoterics may be applied quite easily at home or away from home. The "Bach Flower Therapy" which became popular during the middle of the 20th century is a combination of several essences. It was developed based on the recipe for success, "Heal Thyself" of Edward Bach, MD, the English immunologist and bacteriologist (1886-1936). Already before World War II, he recommended, with success, a varying mixture of 38 flowers from medicinal plants for patients with psychosomatic and painful complaints to stimulate the physical healing powers within their own bodies: "Encourage the body's own potential to look after itself by helping to restore a more positive outlook in times of emotional change". With such a strengthening of their own physical and emotional powers on a natural basis, people are surely much more able to overcome anxiety, depression and pain. At the same time, this stabilises the continu-

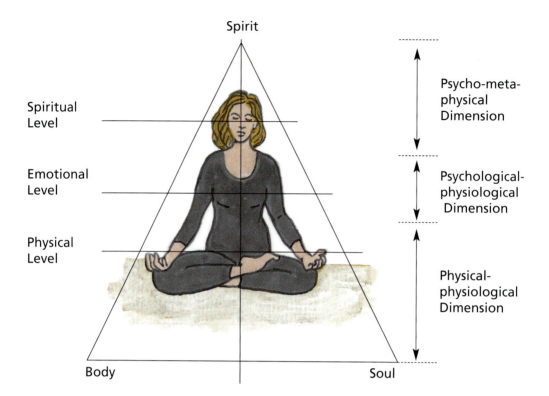

Figure 37:

The Balance between Body and Soul.

ously fluctuating relationship woven between spirit, soul and body. As a rule, almost all natural and alternative healing methods may be used in combination, without any damaging side effects. Ethereal oils, juices, and salves such as those mentioned here as examples, also offer, in combination with alternative measures, valuable building blocks for a healthy well-being. They help to safely reduce the taking of industrially-manufactured medicines which, in spite of their beneficial effects, unfortunately over the long run, often also have damaging side effects. Obviously, the relaxation procedures from massage to meditation also belong to these building blocks for a healthy well-being. They can support or even strengthen the healing powers of nature. Virtually all important health reformers, who parallel to conventional medicine, developed alternative healing methods, such as Franz Anton Mesmer, Sebastian Kneipp (1821-1897) or Edward Bach, wanted to stimulate the inherent resistance of the human body by means of natural, harmless therapies.

The conclusion may then be drawn that natural healing procedures should be used first for incipient or chronic pain. Here too, however, as with any medical therapy, it is important to carefully observe the course of an illness, to administer the correct dosage, and to monitor success or failure. Once again, to quote the Greek physician, Hippocrates, who proved in his writings that in every medicine there is a healing as well as a poisonous effect. Since antiquity therefore, the first commandment of ethics for the medical profession says, in Latin "Nil nocere!" ("Do no harm!").

The starting point of every treatment, whether through the healing powers of nature or with conventional medicine, is again always the plausible thought that often a painful illness that

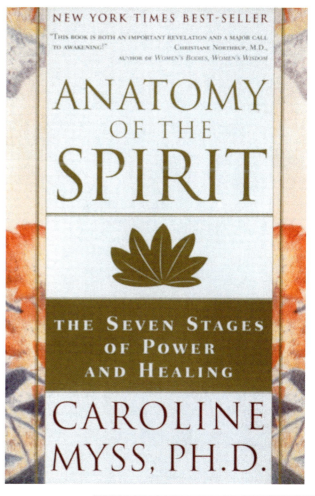

Figure 38:

Title page of the American bestseller by Caroline Myss: Anatomy of the Spirit, published in 1996 in the USA.

is not caused by an infection may actually be caused by physical or emotional disharmony. If this phenomenon is consciously known and observed, mental, meditative and spiritual efforts can be directed towards reducing pain and suffering, with the aim of restoring the balance between body and soul (Figure 37). This also means, however, that medical research should occupy itself more than ever with psycho-neuro-immunology, the science of the combined effects of immunology with the nerve and hormone systems. The influence of self-healing substances within the human body deserves further elucidation. More and more research on these abilities of self-healing, dormant in our body, and the various possibilities of reinforcing them, has been carried out during the last two decades. As a matter of course, the American Caroline Myss also integrates the great religions into her health philosophy in her very readable book, "Anatomy of the Spirit. The Seven Stages of Power and Healing" (1996, Figure 38). She writes typically enough: "The universal jewel within the four major religions is that the Divinity is locked into our biological system in seven stages of power".

Promoting health through spiritual, natural healing and alternative ways and means can surely prevent the pain which may be a part of every illness. A further methodical treatment group for illnesses closely associated with pain is illustrated by physical therapy such as massage, physiotherapy, balneotherapy and thermotherapy. They are belonging to a large number of pain killers, which today are enjoying a renaissance.

Figure 39:

Three different illness scenes in the ward of a hospital around 1605.
Floating over the ward is an angel holding high a medallion which contains a face with a distorted expression.

Copperplate about 1605.

Privately owned

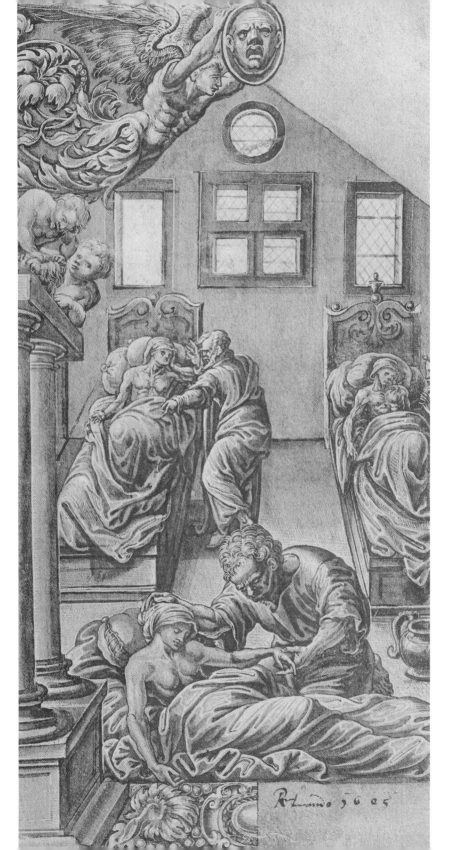

SELECTED LITERATURE

Pain: Diagnosis and Therapy
General

Anschütz, Heinrich Felix: Indikation zum ärztlichen Handeln. Lehre, Diagnostik, Therapie, Ethik. Berlin, Heidelberg and New York 1982.

Auersperg, Alfred: Schmerz und Schmerzhaftigkeit. Berlin, Göttingen and Heidelberg 1963.

Baar, Hugo A. and Hans Ulrich **Gershagen**: Schmerz, Schmerzkrankheit, Schmerzklinik. Berlin, Heidelberg and New York 1974.

Bacon, Douglas R., Vijayalakshmi **Reddy** and Orville T. **Murphy**: Regional anaesthesia and Chronic Pain Management in the 1920s and 1930s. Regional anaesthesia 20 (1995), vol. 3, p. 185-192.

Bäker, Bernard A. and Fritz **Janssen**: Schmerzen und wie man sie behebt. Therapie für jedermann. Munich 1986.

Berg, Frans van den (ed.): Angewandte Physiologie. Bd. 4: Schmerzen verstehen und beeinflussen. Stuttgart 2003.

Besson, Jean-Marie: Der Schmerz. Neue Erkenntnisse und Therapien. Munich 1994.

Blasius, Wilhelm: Wesen, Geschichte und Behandlung des menschlichen Schmerzes. Deutsches Ärzteblatt 75 (1978), vol. 37, p. 2094-2096 u. vol. 38, p. 2164-2167 and vol. 39, p. 2239-2241.

Bohnhorst, Brigitte: Leben mit chronischem Schmerz. Munich 1997.

Bonica, John J.: Clinical Applications of Diagnostic and Therapeutic Nerve Blocks. Springfield 1959.

Bonica, John J.: Management of Pain. 2 Volumes. Philadelphia 1953.

Brena, Steven F.: Chronic Pain: America's Hidden Epidemic. New York 1978.

Brune, Kay, Antje **Beyer** and Michael **Schäfer**: Schmerz. Pathophysiologie - Pharmakologie - Therapie. Berlin 2001.

Fields, Howard L.: Pain. New York 1989.

Flagg, Paluel J.: The Art of Anaesthesia. 7th edition Philadelphia 1947.

Flor, Herta: Psychobiologie des Schmerzes. Bern, Göttingen and Toronto 1991.

Gerhardt, Günter and Julia **Pross**: Schmerzen: Nicht unterdrücken, sondern behandeln. Stuttgart 2003.

Goldscheider, Alfred: Das Schmerzproblem. Berlin 1920.

Gutjahr, Peter (ed.): Schmerz bei Kindern. Schmerztherapie in Arztpraxis und Krankenhaus. Stuttgart 2000.

Hackenthal, Eberhard and R. **Wörz** (eds.): Medikamentöse Schmerzbehandlung in der Praxis. Stuttgart and New York 1985.

Hammer, Claus and Venanz **Schubert** (eds.): Chronische Erkrankungen und ihre Bewältigung. Starnberg 1993.

Handwerker, Hermann O.: Einführung in die Pathophysiologie des Schmerzes. Berlin 1998.

Hardy, James Daniel, Harold G. **Wolff** and Helen **Goodell**: Pain Sensations and Reactions. Baltimore 1952.

Hartmann, Fritz: Die Sprachen der Schmerzen. Der Schmerz 12 (1998), vol. 5, p. 317-322.

Hartmann, Fritz: Teil und Ganzes. Zur Anthropologie des Schmerzes. In: **Eich**, Wolfgang (ed.): Psychosomatische Rheumatologie. Berlin, Heidelberg and New York 1991, p. 7-31.

Janzen, Rudolf, Wolf D. **Keidel**, Albert **Herz** and Carl **Streichele** (eds.): Schmerz. Grundlagen – Pharmakologie – Therapie. Stuttgart 1972.

Keeser, Wolfgang and M. **Bullinger**: Psychologische Verfahren bei der Behandlung von Schmerzen. In: **Pongratz**, Wolf (ed.): Therapie chronischer Schmerzzustände in der Praxis. Berlin, Heidelberg and New York 1985, p. 42-105.

Kieser, Werner: Ein starker Körper kennt keinen Schmerz. Gesundheitsorientiertes Krafttraining nach der Kieser-Methode. New edition Munich 2003.

Klingler, D. and B. **Kepplinger**: Schmerzkliniken - Schmerzambulanzen - Organisationsformen und Strukturen. In: **Bergmann**, Hans (ed.): Moderne Schmerzbehandlung. Wien, Munich and Berlin 1984, p. 44-50.

Liebeskind, John C. and Marcia L. **Meldrum**: John J. Bonica, World Champion of Pain. In: **Jensen**, Troels S., Judith A. **Turner** and Zsuzsanna **Wiesenfeld-Hallin** (eds.): Proceedings of the 8th World Congress on Pain. (Progress in Pain Research and Management; Bd. 8). Seattle, WA 1997, p. 19-32.

Melzack, Ronald: The Puzzle of Pain. Harmoudsworth 1973.

Meyer, Wolfgang: Die Venenpunktion als Schmerzerlebnis. Med. Diss. Frankfurt a.M. 1979.

Michaelis, Adolf Alfred: Der Schmerz, ein wichtiges diagnostisches Hilfsmittel. Eine Schmerz-Theorie. Leipzig 1905.

Miller, Andrew: Ingenious Pain. London 1997.

Nauck, Friedemann and Eberhard **Klaschik**: Schmerztherapie. Kompendium für Ausbildung und Praxis. Stuttgart 2002.

Schmerz. (Du, Zeitschrift für Kunst und Kultur 19 (1959), vol. 2 = No. 216). Zürich 1959.

Seefeldt, Dieter (ed.): Schmerz als psychosoziales Problem. Potsdam 1998.

Sherrington, Charles Scott: On the proprio-ceptive system, especially in its reflex aspect. Brain 29 (1906), p. 467-482.

Smith, W. Lynn, Harold **Merskey** and Steven C. **Gross** (eds.): Pain. Meaning and Management. New York and London 1980.

Sternbach, Richard A.: Pain Patients. Traits and Treatment. New York, San Francisco and London 1974.

Strian, Friedrich: Chronischer Schmerz. In: **Hammer**, Claus and Venanz **Schubert** (eds.): Chronische Erkrankungen und ihre Bewältigung. Starnberg 1993, p. 131-168.

Strian, Friedrich: Schmerz. Ursachen, Symptome, Therapien. Munich 1996.

Szasz, Thomas: Pain and Pleasure. A Study of Bodily Feelings. 2nd ed. New York 1988.

Thiele-Dohrmann, Klaus: Schmerz. Was Leiden lehren kann. Munich 1989.

Thomas, Richard: Pain. The Complete Conventional and Alternative Guide to Treating Chronic Pain. Pleasantville, N.Y. 1999.

Waldvogel, Herman Hans: Analgetika, Antinoziceptiva, Adjuvanzien. Handbuch für die Schmerzpraxis. 2nd ed. Berlin, Heidelberg and New York 2001.

Wall, Patrick David: Defeating Pain: The War Against a Silent Epidemic. New York 1991.

Werner, Ulf: Alarmsignal Schmerz. Seelische Ursachen von Schmerzen verstehen und behandeln. Stuttgart 2004 .

Zenz, Michael and Ilmar **Jurna** (eds.): Lehrbuch der Schmerztherapie. Stuttgart 1993.

Zimmermann, Manfred and Hermann Otto **Handwerker** (eds.): Schmerz. Konzepte und ärztliches Handeln. Berlin, Heidelberg and New York 1984.

Zimmermann, Manfred and Hanne **Seemann**: Der Schmerz. Ein vernachlässigtes Gebiet der Medizin? Defizite und Zukunftsperspektiven in der Bundesrepublik Deutschland. Berlin and Heidelberg 1986.

History of Pain Sensation and Combating Pain in Medicine

Burger, Christof: Die Schmerzbekämpfung in der spanischen Chirurgie (1814-1868). Diss. Cologne 1988.

Dieffenbach, Johann Friedrich: Der Aether gegen den Schmerz. Berlin 1847.

Delingat, Almut: Die Geschichte der Anästhesiologie in Deutschland. Diss. Cologne 1975.

Goldscheider, Alfred: Ueber den Schmerz in physiologischer und klinischer Hinsicht. After a lecture at the Berlin Military Medical Society on 22nd January 1894. Berlin 1894.

Handwerker, Hermann O. and Kay **Brune** (eds.): Deutschsprachige Klassiker der Schmerzforschung. Heidelberg 1987.

Karger-Decker, Bernt: Besiegter Schmerz. Geschichte der Narkose und der Lokalanästhesie. Leipzig 1984.

Keys, Thomas E.: Die Geschichte der chirurgischen Anaesthesie. Berlin 1968.

Killian, Hans: 40 Jahre Narkoseforschung. Erfahrungen und Erlebnisse. Tübingen 1964.

Kuhlen, Franz-Josef: Zur Geschichte der Schmerz-, Schlaf- und Betäubungsmittel in Mittelalter und früher Neuzeit. (Quellen und Studien zur Geschichte der Pharmazie; Bd. 19). Stuttgart 1983.

Mann, Ronald D. (ed.): The History of the Management of Pain. From Early Principles to Present Pain. New Jersey 1988.

Michler, Markwart: Zur Entstehung des medizinischen Schmerzbegriffes. Orthopädische Praxis 15 (1979), p. 347-350.

Morris, David B.: The Culture of Pain. Los Angeles 1991.

Pasch, Thomas and Christoph **Mörgeli** (eds.): 150 Jahre Anästhesie. Narkose, Intensivmedizin, Schmerztherapie, Notfallmedizin. Wiesbaden 1997.

Robinson, Victor: Victory over Pain. New York 1946.

Rodegra, Heinrich and Hans-Wilhelm **Schreiber**: Schmerz im Paradigmawandel der Medizin. Geschichte des Schmerzes - Philosophie - Kultur - Weltanschauung. In: **Beck**, Helge, Eike **Martin**, Johann

Motsch and Jochen **Schulte am Esch** (eds.): Schmerztherapie. Stuttgart and New York 2002, p. 3-7.

Rupreht, Joseph, Marius Jan van **Lieburg**, John Alfred **Lee** and Wilhelm **Erdmann**: Anaesthesia. Essays on Its History. Berlin 1985.

Sauerbruch, Ferdinand and Hans **Wenke**: Wesen und Bedeutung des Schmerzes. Berlin 1936.

Schadewaldt, Hans: Geschichte der Schmerzbehandlung. Medizinische Welt 31 (1980), vol. 36, p. 1277-1279.

Schipperges, Heinrich: Vom Wesen des Schmerzes (1984). In: **Sokolow**, Aleksander and Roman **Kudella**: Schmerzlosigkeit. Zwei Arbeiten zur Geschichte der Anästhesie. (Kölner medizinhistorische Beiträge; 52). Cologne 1989, p. 1-23.

Schüttler, Jürgen (ed.): 50 Jahre Deutsche Gesellschaft für Anästhesiologie und Intensivmedizin. Tradition & Innovation. Berlin and Heidelberg 2003.

Seeman, Bernhard: Über den Schmerz. Geschichte der Schmerzbekämpfung. Heidelberg 1965.

Smith, W. D. A.: Under the Influence. A History of Nitrous Oxide and Oxygen Anaesthesia. London 1982.

Walser, Hans H.: Zur Einführung der Äthernarkose im deutschen Sprachgebiet im Jahre 1847. Aarau 1957.

Zinganell, Klaus: Anaesthesie – historisch gesehen. Berlin 1987.

Pain as a Phenomenon of Cultural History

Azoulay, Isabelle: Schmerz. Die Entzauberung eines Mythos. Berlin 2000.

Bien, Helmut M., Ulrich **Giersch**, Thomas **Gubig** and Sebastian **Köpcke** (eds.): Schmerz laß nach. Drogerie-Werbung der DDR. Ausst.-Kat. ed.: Deutsches Hygiene-Museum Dresden. Berlin 1992.

Engelhardt, Dietrich von: Krankheit, Schmerz und Lebenskunst. Munich 1999.

Farin, Michael (ed.): Lust am Schmerz. Texte und Bilder zur Flagellomanie. Munich 1991.

Farin, Michael (ed.): Phantom Schmerz. Quellentexte zur Begriffsgeschichte des Masochismus. Munich 2003.

Hüper, Christa: Schmerz als Krankheit. Die kulturelle Deutung des chronischen Schmerzes und die politische Bedeutung seiner Behandlung. (Mabuse-Verlag Wissenschaft; 12). Frankfurt a.M. 1994.

Jünger, Ernst: Über den Schmerz. In: **Jünger**, Ernst: Blätter und Steine. Hamburg 1934.

Kurthen, Martin: Der Schmerz als medizinisches und philosophisches Problem. Anmerkungen zur Spätphilosophie Ludwig Wittgensteins und zur Leib-Seele-Frage. Würzburg 1984.

Le Breton, David: Schmerz. Eine Kulturgeschichte. Zürich 2003.

Lenz, Siegfried: Über den Schmerz. Munich 2000.

Lewis, Clive S.: Über den Schmerz. Cologne and Olten 1954.

Pöppel, Ernst: Lust und Schmerz. Grundlagen menschlichen Erlebens und Verhaltens. Berlin 1982.

Scarry, Elaine: The Body in Pain. The Making and Unmaking of the World. New York 1985.

Schmerz beiseite. Wunder der Medizin. (Spiegel spezial; No. 7). Hamburg 1998.

Weizsäcker, Viktor von: Schmerzen. Stücke einer medizinischen Anthropologie. Die Kreatur 1 (1926-1927), p. 315-335.

Naturopathic Methods of Combating Pain

Bach, Edward: Heal Thyself. An Explanation of the real Cause and Cure of Disease. Saffron Waldon 1931 (1987).

Gattefossé, René-Maurice: Aromatherapie. Aarau 1994.

Gattefossé, René-Maurice: Gattefossé's aromatherapy. The first book on aromatherapy. Ed. by Robert B.

Tisserand. Saffron Walden 1993.

Haferkamp, Hans (ed.): Naturheilverfahren. Bd. 4: Einführung und Fortbildung. Stuttgart 1955.

Jütte, Robert: Geschichte der Alternativen Medizin. Von der Volksmedizin zu den unkonventionellen Therapien von heute. Munich 1996.

Kluge, Hannelore: Gesundheit aus der Natur-Apotheke. Alte Heilmethoden neu entdeckt. 2 nd. ed., Rastatt 1988.

Kneipp, Sebastian: Meine Wasser-Kur. 37th ed. Kempten 1892.

Kneipp, Sebastian: So sollt ihr leben! Winke und Ratschläge für Gesunde und Kranke zu einer einfachen, vernünftigen Lebensweise und einer naturgemäßen Heilmethode. 185.-190. Tsd. Munich 1928.

Krug, Erich: Lexikon der Naturheilkunde. Revised and edited by Joachim Moerchel. Heidelberg 1989.

Kursbuch Schmerz. Ursachen, Medikamente, Behandlungsmethoden der Schul- und Alternativmedizin. Cologne 1999.

Lassner, Jean: Akupunktur-Hypnose: Alternativen für die Zukunft? Frankfurt/M. 1976.

Lawless, Julia: Aromatherapie. Ätherische Öle für Körper und Geist. Cologne 1999.

Lust, Benedict: Die Jungmühle. Das Bad der Blutwäsche. Ahrensburg 1968.

Lust, Benedict: Zone therapy. Relieving pain and sickness by nerve pressure. Reprint of 1928 ed. New York 1980.

Melchart, Dieter und Hildebert **Wagner** (eds.): Naturheilverfahren. Grundlagen einer autoregulativen Medizin. Stuttgart 1993.

Natürliche Heilmethoden. Homöopathie, Aromatherapie, Heilsteine, Hausmittel. Bath 2003.

Peck, Connie: Schmerz laß nach! Selbsthilfe bei chronischen Schmerzen. Reinbek bei Hamburg 1990.

Pain and Art

Bader, Alfred: Künstler-Tragik. Karl Stauffer - Vincent van Gogh. Basle 1932.

Bergdolt, Klaus and Dietrich von **Engelhardt** (eds.): Schmerz in Wissenschaft, Kunst und Literatur. (Schriften zu Psychopathologie, Kunst und Literatur; 6). Hürtgenwald 2000.

Borggrefe, Heiner and Vera **Lüpges**: Glanz und Schmerz. Cologne paintings in the Wallraf-Richartz-Museum. Cologne 1998.

Drucker, Michel (ed.): Renoir. Paris 1955.

Eggum, Arne, Gerd **Woll** and Marit **Lande**: Munch im Munch-Museum Oslo. Berlin 1998.

Escholier, Raymond: Henri Matisse. Sein Leben und sein Schaffen. Zürich 1958.

Hammacher, Abraham Marie: Vincent van Gogh. Selbstbildnisse. (Werkmonographien zur bildenden Kunst in Reclams Universal-Bibliothek; Nr. 53). Stuttgart 1960.

Hammacher, Abraham Marie: Vincent van Gogh. Genius and Disaster. New York 1985.

Herrera, Hayden: Frida Kahlo. Malerin der Schmerzen. Rebellin gegen das Unabänderliche. Bern, Munich and Vienna 1983.

Kahlo, Frida: The Diary of Frida Kahlo. An intimate self-portrait. Introduction by Carlos Fuentes. Essay and commentaries by Sarah M. Lowe. New York 1995.

Meier-Græfe, Julius: Auguste **Morris**, David B.: Krankheit und Kultur. Plädoyer für ein neues Körperverständnis. Munich 2000. Renoir. Munich 1911.

Miketta, Gaby: Wie die Seele den Körper heilt. Focus (2003), No. 38, p. 94-104.

Morris, David B.: Illness and Culture in the Postmodern Age. Berkeley and London. 1998.

Murken, Axel Hinrich: Leid, Schmerz und Tod. Die Schattenseiten des Lebens im Spiegel der spanischen Kunst des 17. Jahrhunderts. Die Waage. 42 (2003), p. 32-37.

Nizon, Paul (ed.): Van Gogh in seinen Briefen. Frankfurt am Main 1977.

Prignitz-Pode, Helga, Salomon **Grundberg** und Andrea **Kettenmann** (eds.): Frida Kahlo. Das Gesamtwerk. Frankfurt am Main 1988.

Schneede, Uwe M.: Edvard Munch. Das kranke Kind. Arbeit an der Erinnerung. Frankfurt am Main 1984.

Svenæus, Gösta: Edvard Munch. Das Universum der Melancholie. (Publications of the New Society of Letters at Lund; 58). Lund 1968.

Zell, Andrea: Valie Export. Inszenierung von Schmerz: Selbstverletzung in den früheren Aktionen. Berlin 2000.

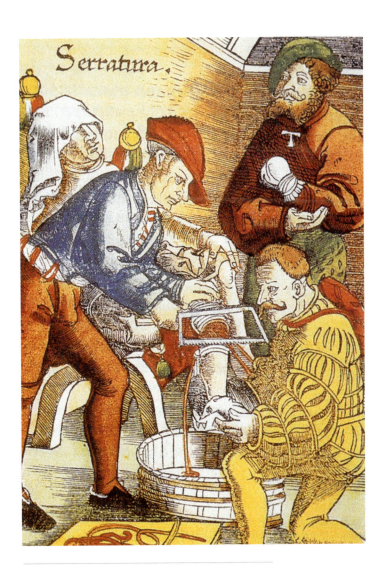

Figure 40:
Illustration of a lower leg amputation in a southern German hospital of the Antonites. A white cloth has been placed over the eyes of the patient who became unconscious due to the pain.

From: Hans von Gersdorff: Feldtbuch der Wundtarzney, Straßburg 1517.

REGISTER OF NAMES

- Achilles, hero of Greek mythology, page 12
- Adam, page 9
- Aesculapius (Asklepios), page 10, 13, 14, 55, 56, 57, 58
- Almodovar, Pedro, page 64
- Amphiaros, page 59
- Anschütz, Heinrich Felix, page 50
- Apollo, page 36, 56, 57
- Archinos, page 59

- Bach, Edward (1886 - 1936), page 71, 73
- Baudelaire, Charles (1821 - 1867), page 33
- Benson, Herbert, page 55, 57
- Bergmann, Ernst von (1836 - 1907), page 2, 24
- Bier, August (1861 - 1949), page 25
- Bigelow, Henry Jacob (1818 - 1890), page 22
- Billroth, Theodor (1826 - 1894), page 29
- Bingen, Hildegard von (1098 - 1179), page 66
- Bonica, John Joseph (1914 - 1994), page 43
- Brandt, Ludwig, page 33
- Brauchle, Alfred (1898 - 1964), page 54, 55
- Braun, Heinrich (1862 - 1934), page 24, 25
- Brena, Steven F., page 45
- Brend'amour, Richard (1831 - 1915), page 29
- Burkhardt, Ludwig (1872 - 1922), page 27

- Camerarius, Joachim (1500 - 1575), page 66
- Canstatt, Karl (1807 - 1850), page 22
- Cosmas (Martyr and doctor, 3rd Century after Christ), page 16

- Damian (Martyr and doctor, 3rd Century after Christ), page 16
- Davy, Humphry (1778 - 1829), page 20
- Descartes, René (1596 - 1650), page 10, 43, 44, 47
- De Quincey, Thomas (1785 - 1859), page 33

- Dieffenbach, Johann Friedrich (1792 - 1847), page 22
- Dioskurides, Pedanios (1st Century B.C.), page 64, 66
- Dräger, Alexander Bernhard (1870 - 1928), page 33

- EFIC (European Federation of the International Association for the Study of Pain Chapters), page 7
- Einhorn, Alfred (1817 - 1917), page 24
- Elisabeth of Hungary, (1207 - 1231), page 38, 39
- Eve, page 9

- Farill, Juan, (1902 - 1973), page 41
- Fischer, Emil (1852 - 1949), page 26
- Freud, Sigmund (1856 - 1939), page 62
- Fuchs, Leonhard (1501 - 1566), page 66
- Furlenmeier, Martin, page 14

- Gersdorff, Hans von (around 1430 - 1529), page 83
- Goldscheider, Alfred (1858 - 1935), page 46, 47
- Grote, Louis Radcliffe (1886 - 1960), page 54
- Grundberg, Salomon, page 41
- Gurlt, Ernst Julius (1825 - 1899), page 27

- Haller, Albrecht von (1708 - 1777), page 46
- Hardy, James D., page 50
- Harvey, William (1578 - 1657), page 10
- Henry II (973 - 1024), page 16, 17
- Herzog, Rudolf (1871 - 1953), page 57
- Hinckley, Robert, (1853 - 1941), page 20
- Hippocrates (460 - 375 B.C.), page 9, 10, 31, 54, 55, 59, 66, 73
- Hoffmann, Felix (1868 - 1946), page 32
- Hogenberg, Abraham (17th century), page 53
- Hygieia, page 14

- Jaspers, Karl (1883 - 1969), page 35
- Jesus Christus († around 30 after Christ), page 8

- John of God (1495 - 1550), page 39
- Jordaens, Jacob (1593 - 1678), page 36, 39

- Kahlo, Frida (1910 - 1954), page 40, 41
- Kettenmann, Andrea, page 41
- Kneipp, Sebastian (1821 - 1897), page 73
- Kuhn, Franz (1866 - 1929), page 29, 31
- Kulenkampff, Dietrich (1880 - 1967), page 41

- Labat, Gaston (1876 - 1934), page 43
- Laocoon (priest of Troja in Greek mythology), page 35, 36
- Larrey, Jean-Dominique (1766 - 1842), page 18, 20
- Leopold (son of Queen Victoria of Great Britain), page 23
- Leriche, René (1839 - 1955), page 41

- Matthioli, Pietro Andrea (1500 - 1577), page 66, 67
- Mayo, Charles (1865 - 1939), page 43
- Melzack, Roland, page 11
- Mering, Joseph von (1849 - 1908), page 26
- Mesmer, Franz Anton (1734 - 1815), page 19, 73
- Mikulicz-Radecki, Johann von (1850 - 1905), page 27
- Morpheus, page 11, 33
- Murillo, Bartolomé Esteban (1617 - 1682), page 39
- Murken, Axel Hinrich, page 8
- Murken, Christa, page 62
- Myss, Caroline, page 73, 74

- Napoleon (1769 – 1821), page 18
- Nicolaus (11th century), page 17

- Oré, Pierre-Cyprien (1828 - 1889), page 27

- Patrokles (hero of Greek mythology), page 12
- Priestley, Joseph (1733 - 1804), page 20
- Prignitz-Pode, Helga, page 41
- Prometheus (hero of Greek mythology), page 9, 36, 37, 39

- Redard, Camille (1841 - 1910), page 27
- Riemenschneider, Tilman (around 1460 - 1531), page 17
- Rousseau, Henri (1844 - 1910), page 61, 62
- Sauerbruch, Ferdinand (1875 - 1951), page 35, 45
- Schimmelbusch, Curt (1860 - 1895), page 23, 24, 27, 29
- Schleich, Carl Ludwig (1859 - 1922), page 23
- Seligmann, Adalbert Franz (1852 – 1945), page 29
- Sertürner, Friedrich Wilhelm (1783 - 1841), page 10, 33
- Simpson, James Young (1811 - 1870), page 22
- Skarbina, Franz (1849 - 1910), page 2
- Snow, John (1813 - 1858), page 22, 23
- Sosias (Sosiaspainter, 500 B.C.), page 12
- Stone, Edward, (1702 - 1768), page 31

- Uffenbach, Petrus (around 1574 - 1635), page 64, 66

- Velpeau, Alfred-Armand (1795 - 1867), page 13
- Vesal, Andreas (1514 - 1564), page 46
- Victoria (Queen of Great Britain, 1819 - 1901), page 23

- Wall, Patrick David, page 11
- Wenke, Hans, (1903 - 1970), page 35, 45

- Zehme, Werner (1859 - 1912), page 24
- Zeus, page 9

Biography of the Author

The author, Axel Hinrich Murken, MD, PhD, born 1937 in Gütersloh, studied medicine, history of art, history and archaeology.

Graduated as doctor of medicine at Münster University in 1965, medical licence in 1968. Doctorate in philosophy at Bonn University 2001.

Lecturer in history of medicine at Düsseldorf University 1973. Professor and scientific counsellor at the Institute of the History and Theory of Medicine at Münster University 1975-1981.

Appointed Professor of History of Medicine at Aachen University and also Managing Director of the Institute of the History of Medicine and Hospitals on February 5th 1981. Author of several books about history of medicine and hospitals, medical education and in children books, art and medicine.

This book was initiated by the international P.A.I.N. Initiative.
Contact person: Klaus Groth, MD, MPH and Sandra Ambroz
Email: service@pain-initiative.com
More information about the P.A.I.N. Initiative find on **www.pain-initiative.com**

With kind support of

Studies of History of Medicine, Art and Literature. Issue 49
A trademark may be protected even if this is not specifically stated.

Bibliographical Information of the German Library
The German Library (die deutsche Bibliothek) lists this publication in the German National Bibliography (deutsche Nationalbibliographie);
Detailed bibliographical data can be found on http://dnd.ddb.de.

ISBN 3-935791-11-9

It is not allowed to photocopy or record this book or parts of it without the express permission of the publishers.

© 2004 by Verlag Murken-Altrogge
52134 Herzogenrath, Germany